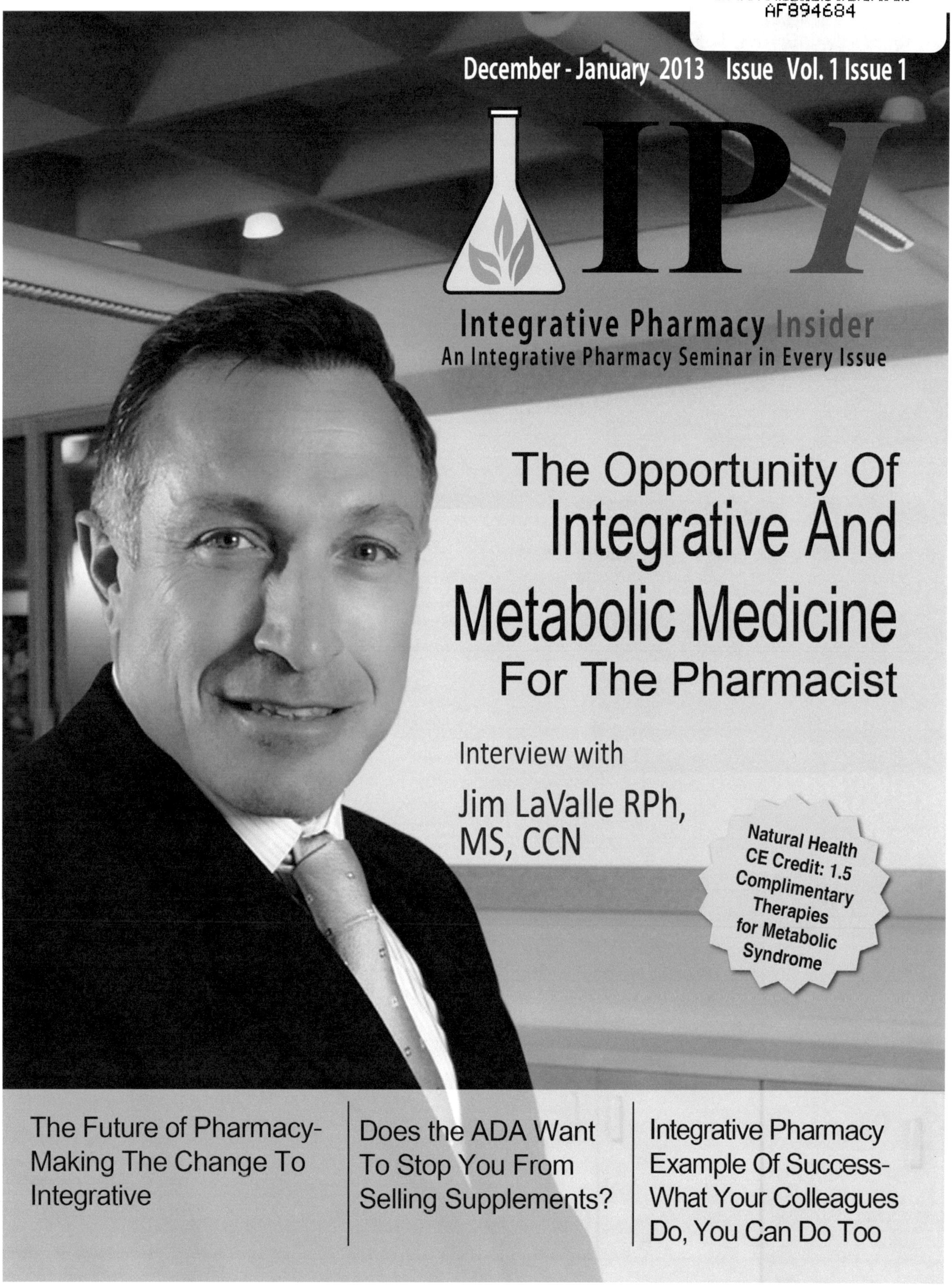

December - January 2013 Issue Vol. 1 Issue 1

IPI

Integrative Pharmacy Insider

An Integrative Pharmacy Seminar in Every Issue

The Opportunity Of Integrative And Metabolic Medicine For The Pharmacist

Interview with

Jim LaValle RPh, MS, CCN

Natural Health CE Credit: 1.5 Complimentary Therapies for Metabolic Syndrome

The Future of Pharmacy- Making The Change To Integrative

Does the ADA Want To Stop You From Selling Supplements?

Integrative Pharmacy Example Of Success- What Your Colleagues Do, You Can Do Too

Rx Letter From The Editor

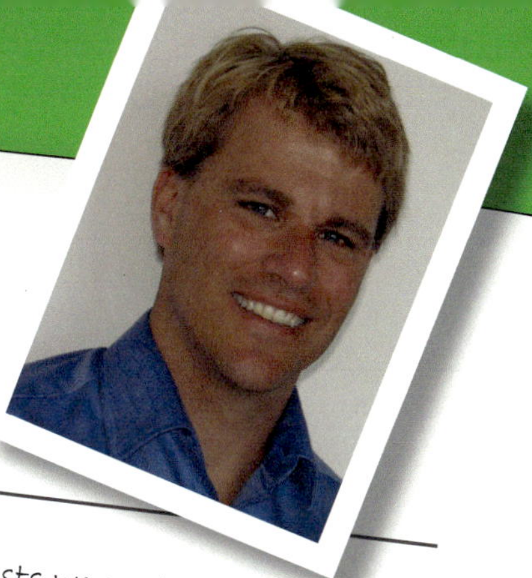

As you read through these pages you will realize that as pharmacists we are in an amazing time of opportunity and growth. It's not just about gainful employment; it's about professional satisfaction and making a difference in peoples lives.

The next few years will not only promise explosive growth within integrative and lifestyle medicine, but as pharmacists we will have the ability to rewrite what it means to be a pharmacist. Integrative medicine has been core to the pharmacy profession, from the beginning, and where many of us are currently capitalizing on nutritional services, consulting, and compounding, things are only just getting started. As you will also see in this and future issues, there are challenges we must be made aware of and we must remain vigilant in protecting our professional and personal sovereignty.

While the folks in Washington continue to bicker over "How much" and "Who is going to pay" there is a better system of medicine, one which recognizes the best of age old traditions and modern discoveries, promotes empowerment and vitality of health, and your customers are looking for this.

My pharmacy career has become one of tremendous satisfaction, but it has not always been that way. When I graduated from pharmacy school in 1994 I was disenchanted with the model of pharmacy, I was nothing more than a drug vendor, watching people get lost on the merry-go-round of drug therapy, treating side-effects with more drugs- it was insanity.

So, I ran away. In the summer of 1995, my wife and I made our exodus from the Philadelphia area and headed west. We ended up in Jackson Hole, Wyoming where for the next eight years I ran a retail pharmacy in a quintessential western ski town.

Like the saying goes, "You can run, but you cannot hide" and that disenchanted model of pharmacy caught up with me, but this time I began to look for a better way of pharmacy.

I always had a penchant for the natural side of things. I was introduced to compounding and realized I could create my own nutritional pharmacy with the credibility of being an official pharmacy, and this proved be the beginning of my journey into integrative pharmacy.

My experience in compounding led me to attain accreditation as a certified clinical nutritionist. The passion we had in what we were doing allowed our compounding/nutritional pharmacy to grow into more of a wellness clinic where we housed integrative practitioners such doctors, nutritionists, skin care specialists and massage therapists. I now have the pleasure of helping others expand their practices and careers in integrative medicine, and realize the more practitioners are involved, the more of an impact we can make.

This first issue of Integrative Pharmacy Insider speaks about the opportunity of integrative and lifestyle medicine, as well as a major area of concern where allopathic medicine has dropped the ball- metabolic syndrome. As you will see such metabolic disorders provide tremendous opportunity for business growth as well as the ability to make a major impact on the health of your community.

Robert Kress, RPh

December - January 2013 Issue Vol. 1 Issue 1

IPI

Integrative Pharmacy Insider

An Integrative Pharmacy Seminar in Every Issue

Table of Contents

Integrative Pharmacy Insider is published 6 times per year; Dec/Jan, Feb/Mar, Apr/May, June/July, Aug/Sept, Oct/Nov

Online subscription access and print editions are available for purchase at **Pharmacistintegrative.com/subscribe.**

What You Need To Know About The American Dietetics' Association And Your Right To Counsel on and Sell Supplements

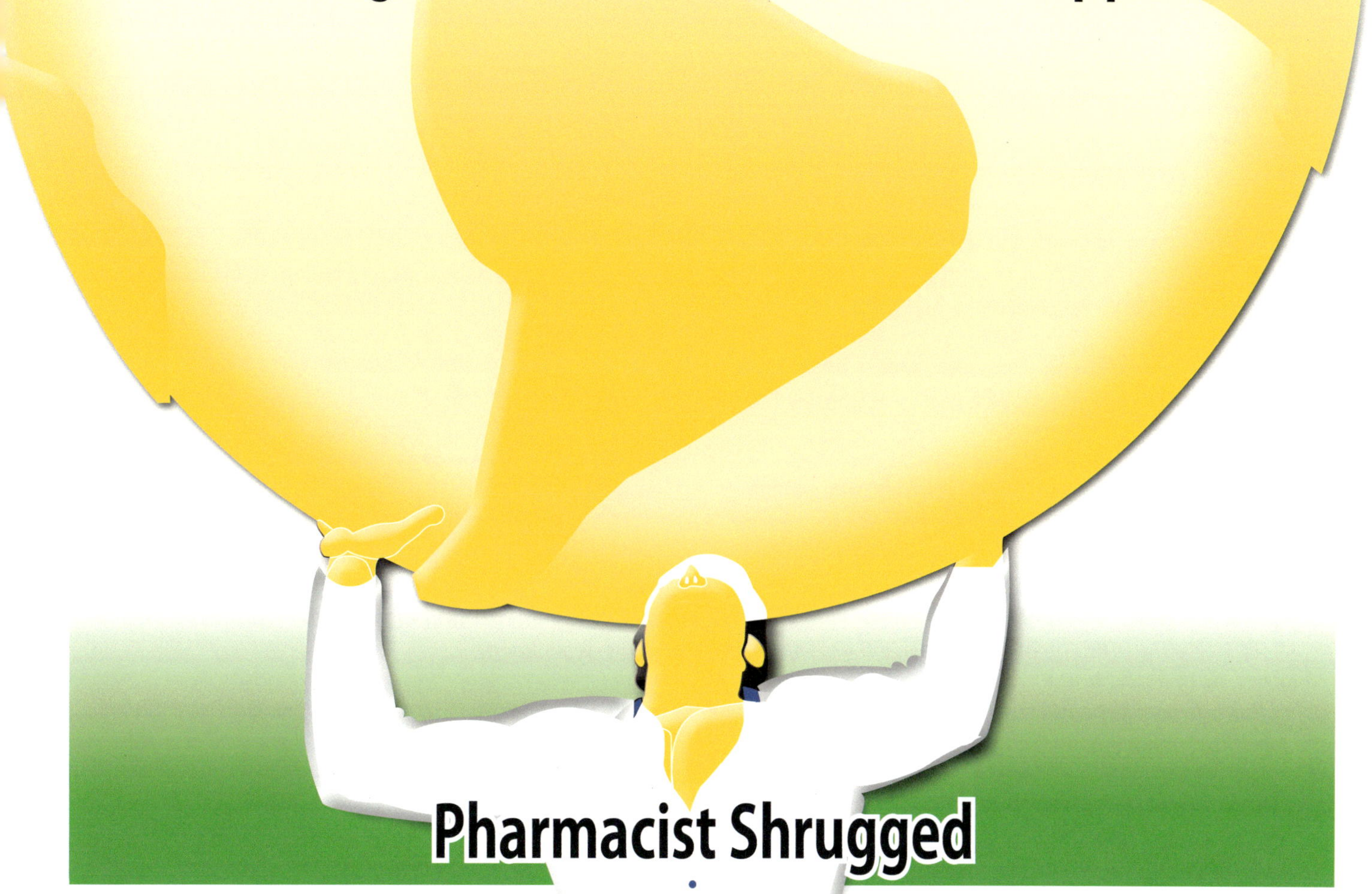

Pharmacist Shrugged

This has become a sordid tale right out of Ayn Rand's Atlas Shrugged. There is a major power grab going on all over the country by the American Dietetics' Association (ADA) with its state run affiliates. At risk is your right to recommend and sell nutritional supplements. And I know, where a common response might be, "that can't affect me, I am a pharmacist", or "that's too farfetched, it will never happen" in some states it is already happening and in others, the laws are written and ready to implement. (Note: The ADA has officially changed its name to the Academy of Nutrition and Dietetics, although for this article I will be referring to them as the ADA)

This topic had initially come to light for me back around 2008 when I was contacted due to my CCN licensure about what was being proposed to take nutrition counseling rights away from anyone who essentially is not a licensed dietician here in my state of Michigan. And my initial response was similar to the above "that can't affect me, I am a pharmacist." Boy was I wrong.

Fast forward to today. Health care professional groups as well as consumers have worked very hard in Michigan to dampen this power grab by the ADA and have made great strides, although the ADA keeps pushing, and other states are at great risk as we speak.

I came across an article written in Forbes titled ***Is the ADA Intentionally Using State Legislatures to Block Alternative Nutrition Providers?*** written by Michael Ellsberg.

Mr. Ellsberg makes note of a Steve Cooksey, a blogger in North Carolina who blogs on his experiences and successful steps he has taken to lose weight, eliminate the need for insulin shots and medication, and he shares these successes with others. (Incidentally, much of what he recommended comes from Mark Sissons Primal Blueprint who has a contribution to this issue.)

Mr. Cooksey then received a disturbing letter from the North Carolina Board of Dietetics/Nutrition. The letter directed Mr. Cooksey to make a series of changes to his blog posts or he would face arrest (according to the NC dietetics licensing statute- one very similar to ones which other states already have or will be moving toward) and up to a month and a half in prison, all for blogging on what worked for him to turn around his health.

Michael Ellsberg addresses the real reason behind the ADA's attempts at such as power grab,.As quoted from his article:

"In these newly-available internal documents, which I quote and outline at length in this article, the American Dietetic Association:

> *Openly discusses creating and using state boards of dietetics/nutrition (including in NC and in every other state in the union) for the **express purpose of limiting market competition for its Registered Dietitian members**.*
>
> *Openly discusses a nation-wide plan of surveilling and reporting private citizens, and particularly all competitors on the market for nutrition counseling, for "harming the public" by providing nutrition information/advice/counseling without a license—through exactly the same means by which Cooksey was reported to the NC Board. Again, for the explicit purpose of limiting marketplace competition.*
>
> *After I read this, I sought to distill down, "what this actually means to the profession of pharmacy and other health care professions". I connected with Michael Stroka, JD, MBA, MS, CNS, CCN, who is the Executive Director of the Certification Board for Nutrition Specialists. Michael is an expert in the legislative issues which concern us, and he has been gracious enough to answer my questions.*

Q: I understand the thing about legislation is often how it is written, and what might not seem to be an issue can in fact be interpreted in many ways and then implemented into law much to the dismay of the populace. Can you share with us some of the concerns in the verbiage of the proposed pieces of legislation and how they can be interpreted into law? Could you also address, what could actually happen if the ADA has its way? For example, will I be able to share with a patient that their statin drug can deplete CoQ10 and recommend that they supplement?

A: Every bill and law is unique, but most have a similar pattern. Below is a typical (very broad) definition of practicing nutrition that appears in most laws or proposed laws:

"Nutrition assessment" means the evaluation of the nutrition needs of individuals or groups using appropriate data to determine nutrient needs or status and make appropriate nutrition recommendations.

"Nutrition counseling" means advising and assisting individuals or groups on appropriate nutrition intake by integrating information from the nutrition assessment.

"Nutrition services for individuals and groups" shall include, but is not limited to, all of the following;

(a) Providing nutrition assessments relative to preventive maintenance or restorative care.

(b) Providing nutrition education and nutrition counseling as components of preventive maintenance or restorative care.

So where exclusionary licensing laws exist (laws stating you must be licensed to do any of these activities), anyone performing any of these actions is treading on the scope of practice of Licensed Dietitian/Nutritionists. That is a violation of the law and considered a criminal act. Remember supplements are classified as "food" under DSHEA, thus anywhere you see "nutrition", supplements are included among the restrictions. In some states, IL for example, supplements are identified as "oral nutrition", and recommending them is specifically included in the licensed practitioner's scope of practice.

In New York for example:

- It appears a pharmacist license in New York does not specifically include nutrition or supplements in its scope of practice. If the scope does include drug-food or drug-supplement interactions, a pharmacist might be safe noting the CoQ10 issue generically, but it is impossible to be certain. Actually recommending the supplement to an individual would seem to be a gray area.

- The ADA has proposed an exclusionary New York nutrition licensing law, that makes the practice of nutrition counseling illegal for all except dietetics license holders and other licensed professionals whose scope of practice includes nutrition/dietetics.

- Thus, pharmacists in New York would be violating the state's nutrition licensing law by recommending supplements tailored to meet a specific individual's health needs.

One important note to keep in mind is that each law has its own language, and it is very hard to generalize. And even then, the language or its interpretation is often gray. It is important to review your state's laws thoroughly, and consult an attorney for interpretation of your circumstances.

Q: I understand that the ADA is proposing "watch dog" policies, such as surveillance of and reporting on private citizens. This sounds like police state tactics, how accurate and true is this?

A: The press has published documents indicating that the ADA is conducting training and otherwise incentivizing its Registered Dietitians to identify and report unlicensed activity.

Anecdotally, we have seen an increase in the number of individuals being sent cease and desist letters and otherwise being pursued by licensing boards.

Q: From a retail point of view, what impact will this make? For example, will retailers be able to carry the products, but if they are not a registered dietician, they cannot recommend or offer any counseling for risk of criminal punishment?

A: Each law is unique. But most contain the following type of exemption from the Licensing Requirement:

"A person from providing general non-medical nutrition information as an operator or employee of a health food store or business that sells health products, including dietary supplements, food, or food materials, or disseminating written nutrition information in connection with the marketing and distribution of those products."

That language is there to permit retail and health food stores to sell food and supplements. based exclusively on general, and generic information about the product. However, that does not allow the 'practice of nutrition.' The laws are quite clear that the acts of those store employees must not cross the line into the practice of nutrition, which essentially means any of these pieces: the assessment of someone's nutrition status, evaluation of their food and supplement needs based on their individual circumstances, and food or supplement recommendations following from that. Thus if a store employee was to gather information about the customer's individual health status, and then recommend supplements based on that, he or she violates the law unless he has a nutrition license or has another license that specifically includes nutrition in its scope.

Q: If these laws were to go into effect, what can the consumer expect as they are searching for answers? For instance, it is well known that competition breeds quality and entrepreneurship; could over-regulation inhibit entrepreneurship and restrict competition, leading to increased costs and decreased levels of service for consumers?

A: Nutrition advice is not the purview of any single profession. It is a toolset used effectively by a great many different types of professionals, including pharmacists. Given our obesity and chronic disease crisis and the fact that nutrition is the most important factor and tool in combatting that crisis, it would be ill-conceived to artificially restrict the ability to provide nutrition advice to solely one particular subset of professionals, ie dietitians. Competition among many qualified groups of professionals to provide nutrition advice would provide greater choice, quality, access, and cost-effectiveness for the public.

Q: I understand that even though the ADA is behind this on a national level, they have infused themselves in the state affiliates, and the impact on pharmacists and other health care professionals will vary from state to state based on the particulars of that state's law. Also the wording is of the pharmacists scope of practice in a given state is key for that profession.. For pharmacists concerned about this (which should be all of them), what do you recommend their next step to be to find out more?

Every pharmacist who provides individualized nutrition or supplement advice should be very concerned.

1. Look up your state's pharmacist scope of practice contained in your licensing law. Your state association can be a good resource for this, but searching "phamacists scope of practice (your state)" is a good place to start.You most likely will need to read the actual rules and regulations to get this information.

2. If your license's scope does not *explicitly* permit you to provide nutrition advice, supplement recommendations, or other tasks you perform, then you are potentially at risk.

3. If so, email us at office@cbns.org with your state, contact info, and scope language, and we can point you in the right direction.

Thank you Michael for helping to identify and clarify the impact these provisions can have on our profession, as well as how they can affect the consumer and the landscape of health care in general.

I think it is clear that this is a very real threat. Each and every state could be impacted differently depending on how the pharmacist's scope of practice is currently written in relationship to nutritional services, as well as the content of the proposed laws which can be unique for each and every state.

You have also given us a clear and simple step by step approach on how to identify the issues which might be challenging our practices, and a direction to go.

We as pharmacists fit perfectly into the nutritional equation due to our knowledge of the relationships between: drug to drug interactions, drug induced nutrient depletions, and drug and nutrient disease state circumstances. It certainly would be a crime to allow speaking from this expertise to be taken away from our profession and the community which our profession serves.

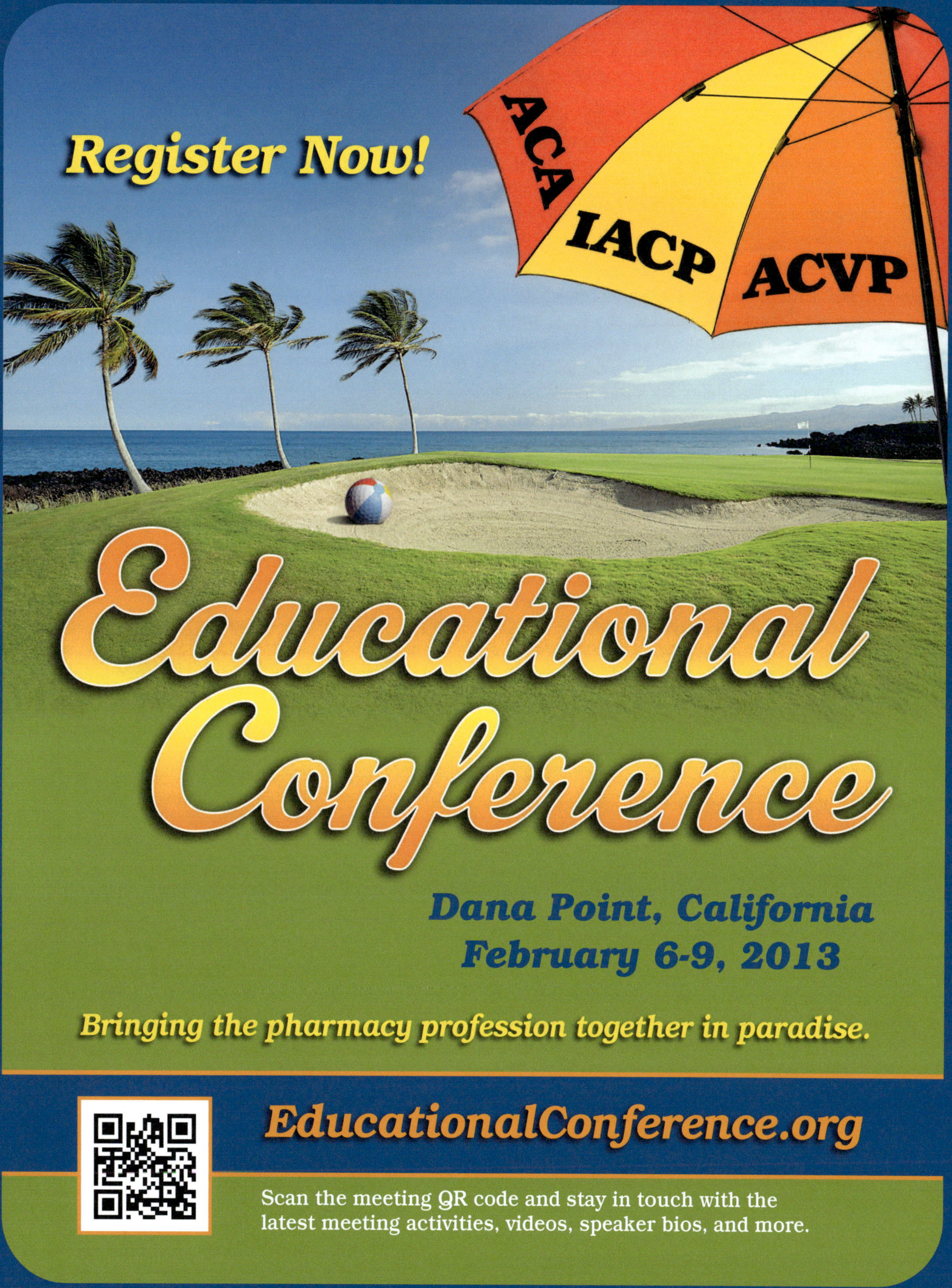

Register Now!
ACA
IACP
ACVP
Educational Conference
Dana Point, California
February 6-9, 2013
Bringing the pharmacy profession together in paradise.
EducationalConference.org
Scan the meeting QR code and stay in touch with the latest meeting activities, videos, speaker bios, and more.

Interview with **Jim LaValle RPh, MS, CCN**

They say if you follow your passion, success will follow, and Jim LaValle RPh, MS, CCN is the perfect example. Jim's passion for helping people through integrative medicine as a practitioner, an educator, and as a consultant has had a tremendous influence on the strength and direction of integrative medicine today.

I was first introduced to Jim during my training for Certification in Clinical Nutrition and like many who experience Jim lecture, I walked away motivated, inspired, and excited about what was awaiting for me in my career. This is why for the first issue of Pharmacist Integrative I can think of no one better to share their expertise on the opportunity of Integrative and Metabolic Medicine for the pharmacist.

Rob: **Jim, I think you are the perfect example of where integrative medicine can take someone in their professional practice, as well as the impact that one can have on integrative medicine. You definitely show how being a pharmacist puts oneself in a perfect position within our medical system; a medical system where prescription drugs play such a large role, and we do have a big need for an integrative approach.**

Jim: Well, yeah, there's no doubt about it. I mean you have to appreciate what a pharmacist can bring into the equation for personalized health and personalized medicine because of our training, so I could not agree with you more.

Rob: **And I think people will see that the opportunities are limitless far beyond what we might perceive in our everyday professional pharmacy environment.**

Jim: Well, you know, I think that if you believe as a pharmacist that your opportunities are limited then that's what's going to come true for you, is that I only can do this. You know, I can only be in a community pharmacy setting and that's it. Gee, I'm not going to be in an independent setting or I can't reach out and compound. I can't reach out and be that clinical practitioner that I thought I could be. Well, yeah, if you believe that, you're right you won't be able to do it. If you really get focused on what you want to accomplish with your pharmacy, you know, your license and your pharmacy training and your pharmacy passion- I mean that's what I call it because I'm passionate about being a pharmacist. You know, I love it. And I think that then the skies open up and then there's nothing but opportunity in front of us over the next 20 years.

Rob: **What brought you to the integrative side of medicine?**

Jim: When I first got out of pharmacy school I got turned on to integrative medicine- and for personal reason. I experienced integrative care from a doctor up in Midway, Ohio and- so then it was interesting. You know, you asked me about limits and where opportunities are, my

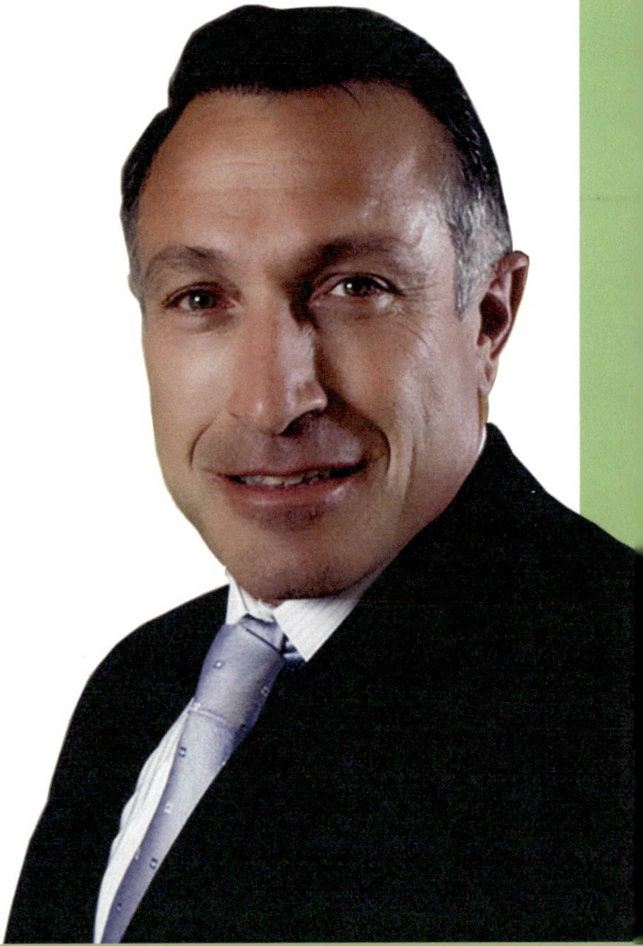

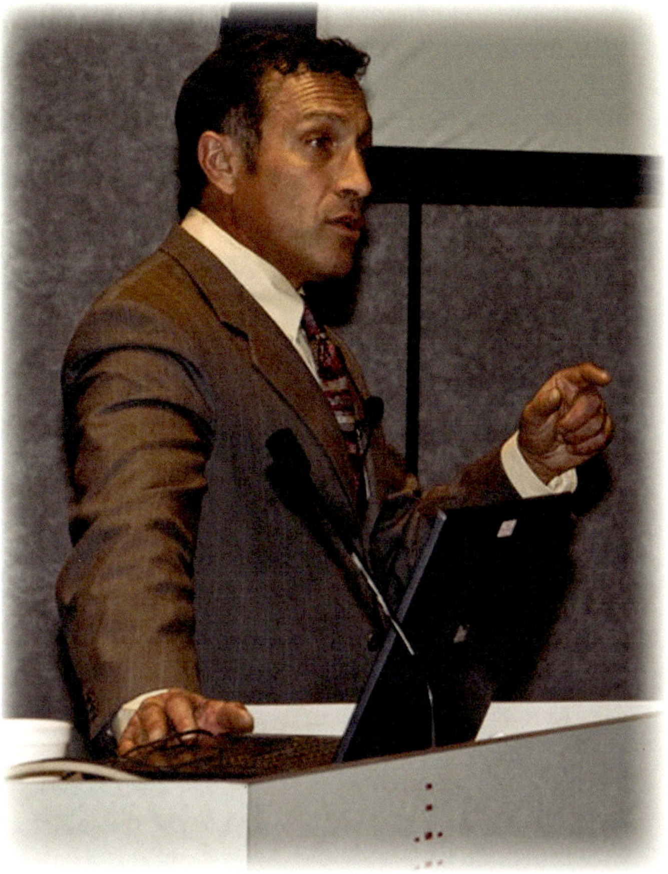

first thought was "Why did I choose pharmacy? How come I didn't go to chiropractic school or osteopathic school or naturopathic school? My gosh, why, why, why?" And then I started to realize that as I looked at integrative medicine and I started to look up all the studies on botanicals coming out of Europe, all the people listed on the studies were in pharmacy.

Rob: Isn't that incredible?

Jim: Yeah. And it was like this bell went off that said, oh my gosh- I could not have been trained better to do what I now do today, you know, virtually thirty years later. I am so grateful that I chose the path I did and I am really grateful for the profession of pharmacy because of it, because I don't think there's a better course of study to understand integrative medicine because it's all cell biology and we have to learn every organ system, every disease state, every kind of drug mechanism. So it was a fantastic training for me.

Rob: So natural medicine actually has core to pharmacy.

Jim: It is core to pharmacy. When I went to pharmacy school, I still had Pharmacognosy. I had Organic Medicinal Chemistry. We had Pharmacy Compounding. We had literally a full year of pharmacy compounding in lab.

You know, I was fortunate that one of my professors was a compounder for Jergens. And we were schooled in the art of pharmacy, in the art and power of natural compounds. And now, as you know, I've taught in pharmacy school for 14 years before I gave it up two years ago and now I'm just teaching as an adjunct faculty at a medical school program. But our students have kind of lost touch with that side of where a lot of these compounds that are still coming from are still from natural products and it's going to get bigger. You know, it's not going away. It's getting bigger in terms of the pipeline. Yeah, you're right. It is our heritage and it is where we're coming from and it is where we're going to.

Rob: You're still teaching with the fellowship? Is that correct?

Jim: Absolutely. Absolutely. I'm very passionate about teaching with the fellowship because it's our ability to reach out and teach thousands of, initially physicians but now other healthcare providers, within the fellowship for Anti-Aging, Regenerative, and Functional Medicine and it's a really rewarding experience because you get people who are kind of unsure, much like yourself, you were compounding and you walked into my facility and you looked back and looked at all the nutrition there and you went, "Holy cow!" I love opening the world up and giving people programs and platforms that they go back, they try on their patient, they come back to me and go, "You know what, that insomnia protocol you gave me, I cannot believe how well that works on all my patients, and I'm getting them off of their drugs and they're feeling better and they're sleeping better." So that is so rewarding working with the fellowship.

Rob: **You mentioned The Fellowship orginated with doctors, but it seems to be the perfect opportunity for pharmacists, don't you agree?**

Jim: Oh, I think fellowship is a great opportunity for pharmacists to get trained and I think it exposes them to a lot of different ideas, a lot of different ways of doing things with practitioners. It gives them a great forum to communicate and connect with other practitioners who are likeminded and I think that's important so you don't feel like you're alone out there. I mean to be quite honest when I started in this, you know, close to 30 years ago, I was in the room where there weren't a lot of doctors in the room and there weren't a lot of pharmacists in the room. And so it made you kind of feel a little isolated. I'm really happy to see now as there is a true sense of fellowship. There is a true sense of people working together and excited about helping people become well and I think that's why the fellowship, in addition to its training and education, is so valuable and it really validates your sense of purpose and your sense of connectiveness to helping people get well.

Rob: **You talked about your number of years in practice. How has the reception changed from the allopathic community over the years?**

Jim: Oh, well, I mean let's just say I went from the red-headed stepchild to the beautiful blond in the room. You know...

When I started teaching at the University of Cincinnati, College of Pharmacy and brought back a course called "A Survey in Natural Medicine," I think a lot of eyebrows were up in the academic setting, but a lot of students flocked to it. And over a period of 15 years it became a very popular course. Students responded beautifully to it because they said, "My god, we're getting questions about this stuff all the time."

And so, you know, over the past 27 year's total, I would say it went from literally me being in fear, I mean if I have to be very honest with you. I mean I literally lived in fear. "Oh my god, am I going to get my door broken down?" I think I'm just doing something good. I explain in a waiver what I'm doing and I'm not practicing medicine and I don't have a tongue depressor down on anyone. I'm doing an interview, I'm looking at what condition they have and I'm making suggestions on what ways they can improve their health. But, you know, 27 years ago, there was no map, there was no model. There was a lot of questions about it. And quite frankly, people's doors were getting broken into and broken down, right? You know, you got the Jonathan Wrights to the world, where they were going in and they were doing some pretty rough stuff. And so, you know, I always was sensitive to the fact that, you know what, there are two ways you could do it: You could be a pioneer, but a lot of times, you know, pioneers end up with arrows on their back. This came about after some pretty deep introspection and when I decided to really move forward in the pharmacy world and that was a real focus to make a conscious effort in pharmacy, you know, work with actually bigger groups like McKesson- I did some things at first with CVS to get my notoriety. So it's, like, wow, you're with a big chain, that means you can work with our independent group like, you know, like a cardinal, and I put together the drug/nutrient depletion groups.

So I strategically started to consult with companies that made me look- "Hey, this guy is legit. You know, he's doing consulting with Roche and Pfizer and AmeriSource and Cardinal Health." And I felt that was important to get credibility and get acceptance even when I went to go and lecture at pharmacy schools to discuss things like drug-induced nutrient depletion which quite honestly, 20 years ago, people were looking at you and going, "Huh? What are you talking about?" And so, it was a very- I could be honest. I was very strategic about making sure that I was evidence-based, that I had a lot of studies behind what I was talking about.

I've been in this business 30 years and finally the opportunities are here. And I would say that the opportunities are here, they're now, they're big. Pharma is interested- I would say medical schools are very interested obviously by University of South Florida's involvement with the Fellowship.

So I think today we have one weak link in this whole process and it's the variability in the quality of the product still and that's an area that I think, you know, look, we just have to talk about it and be open about it. It's an area that needs to be improved. And the industry is exploding and the industry is going to explode even more because it's finally hitting mainstream that people want to be well, they're willing to spend money on being well, and oh by the way, they want their healthcare providers to be involved in keeping them truly well, not just well-checked, not just how good are you taking your medicine, but how do I limit my meds, how do I feel more vital, how do I reduce my weight loss, how do I limit the progression of my condition? The consumer is driving all this, I can tell you right now.

Rob: Can you speak about as far as regulations and policies that we keep seeing knocking at the door of Natural Medicine?

Jim: Well, you know, I think obviously with income and with explosive growth come regulations. It's like there's always regulation with growth and I think that what we need to do on policing regulation we cannot deny access to wellness to consumers, as soon as we legislate restriction- and for example, should it only be dieticians that give recommendations on dietary supplements or diet? Well, I don't know about you but certified diabetic educators and pharmacists have been working with diabetics for the last 60 years and I think it's a huge mistake that we're getting off the right to counsel our patients on diet especially in these areas.

Rob: And that's a very real thing.

Jim: Oh, that's a very real thing. This is very relevant.

Rob: And I think a lot of pharmacists are thinking, "Well, I've got my license. This is only affecting the unlicensed folks."

Jim: That's not the case. That's exactly right. However, dietary supplements are called dietary supplements therefore regulated as a food. If you start seeing legislation where it's "dieticians are the people for food," that means they'll be the people for dietary supplements as well because that's how they're regulated in this country. And you could find yourself out of the ability as a pharmacist to not be able to participate in that other than, you know, being able to do it under a physician's order or under a dietician's order and I think that would be unfortunate when you look at the opportunity to develop programs and platforms for patients that are from the pharmacist's perspective because what I know about pharmacists is they understand drug to drug interaction better, drug/nutrient interaction better, drug disease state interaction better, and I think that what we've done so far is we have not recognized pharmacist as a primary healthcare provide.

On a dietary supplements side, this whole thing of new drug applications or a new dietary ingredient, meaning certain requirements before it can get on the market, is going to be an issue and that we're going to have to be, you know, very- it's going to be harder and harder to get new things out on the market. I think that's reality but there's a lot of GRAS approved or Generally Recognized As Safe ingredients out there that because of new extraction technologies and methodologies we're going to be able to have a large library of nutrients to recommend in the future. And I think that part of it is bright. I think where we need more regulation is we have to ensure the quality of the product.

I saw a study. It's an unpublished study but I saw a study on 28 different bilberries that were on the US market. You know, bilberry extracts. Only two of them actually contained bilberry extracts. So, you know, from my end it's like, look, if they've got a diabetes and they're buying bilberry because they're trying to save their diabetic retinopathy from getting worse or they're trying to prevent diabetic retinopathy, that person deserves the right to buy real bilberry. And if we've got products on the market that aren't real bilberry, that's a problem for me. And so I know that, you know, we have this, we're anti-regulation, I know from the compounding perspective there's always kind of juxtaposition against to some extent with FDA because of the pressure that comes from pharma on, you know, hey, we want pills to be sold that are premade and we know that compounding brings its value on a multitude of levels because of its ability in individualized medications, and you know, from a variety of dosage forms to dosing to pediatric situations, veterinary applications, there's all kinds of ways that compounding brings out value.

And so that's a separate issue and I think we have to be ever vigilant about the compounder's right to treat people as individuals because we're moving to individualized medicine. That's where we're moving. Personalized medicine is where the whole industry is going. And then we have to make sure from a dietary supplements side that we don't get so arrogant that we don't recognize the need to patrol ourselves so that the charlatans and the people that are trying to sell, you know, products as a scam are not getting caught and are not getting reprimanded because that's what they need.

Rob: Speaking of supplements, are there any kind of hot nutrients on your radar right now?

Jim: Well, you know, I think Berberine is a great example, we started tracking Berberine when it was a proprietary ingredient called Flavoxine. This is like seven years ago when I did some studies on looking at lipids on it. And so, you know, Berberine compounds are very interesting because they do have some antimicrobial facts then they have this great kind of metabolic effects where you improve your lipid profile and you also reduce fatty liver. There are a lot of benefits with it.

Even though it's not brand new I think people still don't know about Aged Garlic Extract and I know another study that came out, you know, showing that even the American Heart Association in their newsletters that they send out showed that it may reverse plaque. That's huge for dietary supplement. You know, for the American Heart Association to print that? That's big, right? But nobody is talking about aged garlic, you know? And then of course it can reverse bone mineral density loss which is of course a principal component to corneal calcification and also helps with reduction of fatty liver. So I think Aged Garlic Extract is big because it does a lot of things like that and also works on human trials on it in terms of improving immunity for cold and flu and all those different benefits.

I think Phytosome Curcumin is going to be huge because when people understand that Curcumin just doesn't absorb that well they'll stop, you know, eating so much Curcumin and they'll take something that actually absorbs, and why it's important is it down-regulates so much inflammation in your body systemically. And I'll tell you what, there are athlete's studies on it and there are GI studies on it. Curcumin is beneficial in protecting your kidneys, which if there's a hidden problem that's looming that we're not talking about is the whole issue of Chronic Kidney Disease and Chronic Kidney Intoxication. And you know, even people in our field they don't work on the kidneys enough and this is a major source of problems. And so that's big.

I think Boswellia Phytosome brings a lot to the market. I think it's exciting. I think Evodia Extract is great in terms of fat burning and improving Serotonin production because it up-regulates something called Tryptophan Hydroxylase which is the enzyme that helps you to make Serotonin so, you know, your appetite gets better and it improves uncoupling protein-1 which is, you know, a way that your body finds out how it can burn fat again, right? So, you know, everybody is hot on doing HCG for years. And we did HCG in our clinic as a part of a weight loss program. But, you know, what we quickly found was that a lot of people balloon right back, some people didn't maintain the weight loss, unless you worked on their metabolism. So you could use the HCG to restore the hypothalamus' ability to get to the fat, you know, by signaling. But if you didn't restore all these other aspects to their chemistry typically the weight came back on- and because we researched this pretty thoroughly. And so that's why I think Evodia is so interesting because it opens up those uncoupling proteins and you burn fats.

So I think those are some interesting targets: Aged Garlic, Evodia, Phytosome, Boswellia. You know, obviously the Monoglyceride CoQ10 that I think has shown itself to be the best absorbed Coq10. It's not a well-absorbed compound and you know, so I think that's a big one. There are still a lot of people are believing the marketing hype and not looking at the science of Ubiquinone, instead believe in the hype behind Ubiquinol. And I think it's unfortunate that there's, you know, once again, thrive of marketing over science.

Rob: That's great. I appreciate that. Any last words?

Jim: Last words. I would say that you know what, it is when you called me up and asked me if I would be interested in doing this interview, it was interesting for me, it was a very humbling thing because, you know, I've been so passionate about pharmacy for so many years and it just brought me to full circle, understanding that, you know, you are starting a publication and starting an interaction to get the word out about the value of the independent pharmacist in the integrative care model and for my view, me being able to play a role in helping that gestation with a lot of other people out there in the industry as you know, it's just fantastic. And so, you know, what I would encourage anybody to do is, you know, the thing you do is you follow your passion and if you follow your passion success always follows. It's the way I've always believed in my career was that my biggest passion in life was how can I help the next person. And when I devoted myself to being of service to people that's when it made a difference, when I really wanted to reach out, when I didn't want to ignore someone anymore. Youre an independent pharmacist, you've got 200 people a day walking in that door with a chance for you to change their lives. And it doesn't have to be all-encompassing but you can give them one more step that can help them feel a little bit better, and to me that's what our profession has been all about.

Rob: And with 23,000 independent pharmacies across United States that's a lot of people we can help.

Jim: Let me tell you something. That with 23,000 independent pharmacies across United States we can change U.S. health and we can change a generation of people and I firmly believe that and I'm passionate about that moving forward. So you're absolutely right.

The complete interview, audio and transcript can be downloaded at www.pharmacyunplugged.com

Jim Lavalle's Bio:

Jim LaValle RPH CCN MS. Jim is a nationally recognized clinical pharmacist, author, and educator. He's written over 20 books, including **Cracking the Metabolic Code** and **The Nutritional Cost of Prescription Drugs**, two of my favorites; hundreds of articles, three information databases. He's been named one of the "*50 Most Influential Pharmacists*" by the American Druggist magazine, and the "*2011 Clinician of the Year*" by the Natural Products Association.

Jim has lectured for thousands of healthcare practitioners and consumers all over the world, mainly topics of integrative medicine such drug-induced nutrients depletion and application of natural therapeutics, and has done well over 500 media appearances on radio and TV.

www.jimlavalle.com

jimlavalle@ihr-services.com

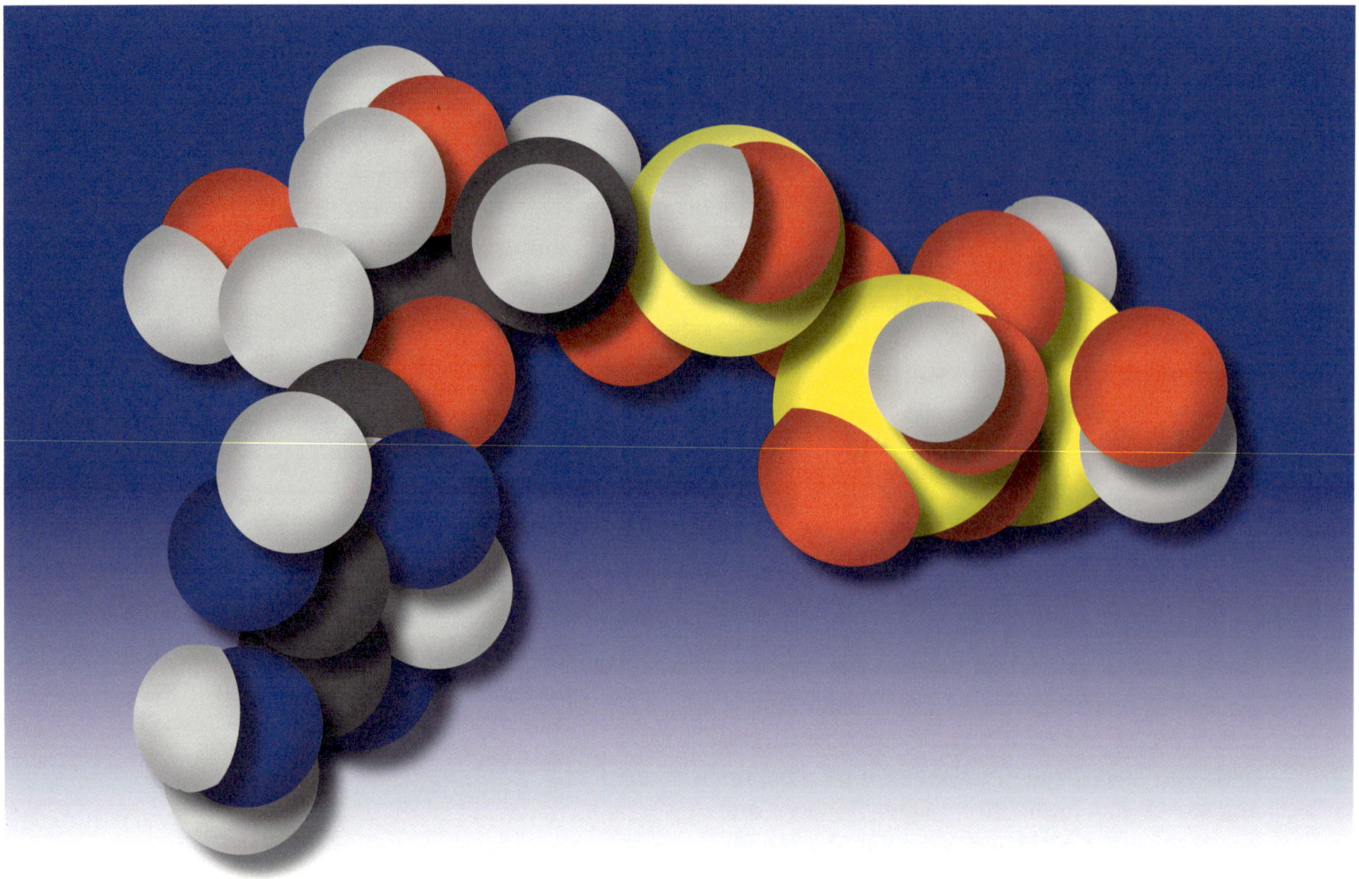

Metabolic Trends- Diabetes

Pharma is Betting On It···Are You?

Much of the growing metabolic syndrome crisis is due to the rising rates of insulin resistance and diabetes. This in fact provides a tremendous opportunity for the independent pharmacy market to help assess, identify, counsel and provide nutritional support to reverse this trend of diabetes rising at such a starling pace.

We as pharmacists are at ground zero when it comes to diabetes. We are where our customers come to once they are diagnosed, and we should be the ones they come to for preventing the disease in the first place.

We have seen more and more pharmacists and staff go down the road of becoming Certified Diabetes Educators, but why wait for the diagnoses of diabetes before we take action? Don't get me wrong, Certified Diabetes Educators are a great resource for patients, especially when diabetes itself can be difficult for many to manage; there is just so much opportunity to take hold of in the realm of pre-diabetes, and insulin resistance.

I hope to see more and more pharmacies instituting their own **Diabetes Prevention Programs** since they have the tools and the access to provide valuable assessments such as Hba1C and even broader based testing services such as those mentioned in the ***"How To Test For Metabolic Syndrome."***

It seems the conversation based on diabetes is all about "what new drugs can we develop to treat the disease" and "how and who is going to pay for it." Shouldn't the conversation be about "let's focus on preventing this very preventable disease"- we have the tools and knowledge to do so, let's just do it.

The numbers of the escalating rates of diabetes, morbidity, mortality and financials are startling:

Type 1 diabetes rose 23% among young people during the first nine years of the 21st century, while type 2 increased by 21%, according to Dr. Dana Dabelea of the University of Colorado in Denver.*

Diabetes contributes to the deaths of more than 230,000 Americans each year. About $174 billion was spent to treat diabetes in the U.S. last year, while chronic diseases in total accounted for about 75% of total health-care spending, according to the ADA.*

The disease is "expanding dramatically" and can even be called a "pandemic," said the head of Novo Nordisk's U.S. business, Jerzy Gruhn. Some models forecast the number of affected people doubling to between 50 million and 55 million by 2025 from 26 million in the U.S. today, he said.*

Jefferies analyst Jeffrey Holford recently told clients that the key diabetes brands and markets will exhibit "sustainable high-single-digit growth," reaching about $54 billion annually by 2020 as the Western population continues to age, obesity rates rise, health-care reform boosts the amount of people who have access to key drugs and experimental therapies come on line.*

As you can see, insulin resistance and diabetes is not only shuttling our healthcare system down an unsustainable road, it is causing Pharma to bet its chips on the diabetes market for the future.

And it's not just Pharma. The diabetes nutritional supplement category has seen explosive growth, sales increasing 50% over the last four years, and forecasts show it will continue to grow at an explosive pace.

"Metabolic syndrome is driver for the next 25 years that I can see, specifically adiposity," said Systems Biosciences' Tim Avila. "Everyone's got it. If it was cancer they'd say it was end of the world. That's the driver. It's bankrupting governments so that's what needs to be fixed."**

The diabetes supplements market has seen impressive growth lately. In 2006, *Nutrition Business Journal* put diabetes supplement sales at $670 million. By 2010 that number reached $1 billion— that's 50 percent growth in four years. **

So where do we go from here?

As you can see, we as pharmacist sit in a very unique position; we are at the cross section of medicine and natural supplements. The future is literally ours to do what we wish with it.

Everyone will attack this differently from the very basic metabolic and sugar support supplements to implementing a full blown Diabetes Prevention Program. I remember as I was a pharmacy intern while in pharmacy school and cough and cold season was just around the corner. The pharmacist I was working with shared with me some sage advice, "get your favorite cough and cold recommendations down now to save you a lot of time when the season hits."

My sage advice to you; the season of metabolic and diabetes crisis is here, decide on your point and shoot blood sugar/metabolic support protocol before opportunity leaves you reacting from your heels.

Next, consider a Diabetes Prevention Program; this can be as basic or intricate as you wish. Here are 4 components which come to mind.

1. Assessment- Whether you consulting on the tests your client brings from the doctor or performing many of the in house diabetes and metabolic tests afforded to us.

2. Supplement Arsenal- Have your favorite supplement protocols on deck.

3. Dietary Recommendations- Even if you feel you are not well versed in recommending dietary food habits, there are a ton of great books on the subject to support individuals with insulin resistance and diabetes.

4. Bonus- Implementing further lifestyle support programs in your practice including but certainly not limited to:
   - Meetings or hosting support groups
   - Presentations and work shops
   - Weight loss programs

The Future of Pharmacy: Making the Change to Integrative

It is common knowledge that the days are gone when you could rely on prescriptions alone to keep your pharmacy thriving. The smart pharmacies are realizing that they are perfectly positioned to expand their expertise and become a closer ally and medical confidante for their patients through an integrative approach.

While change may be difficult, it is the future for the success of your pharmacy. The **Pharmacists OnLine** message for the last eight years has been to inform and encourage our independent pharmacies to be in charge of their destiny, make use of their existing knowledge and expand to attract more customers.

While the integrative approach has long been a success in Europe and Canada, there are many different reasons for the shift to integrative in the U.S. The primary one seems to be aging Baby Boomers that are more receptive to integrative and natural alternative medical aspects. This factor has been combined with the international elevation of global awareness for the overall health attitudes in both personal, earth and energy. When you add the New Millenials to the mix, that have a vast interest in integrative and 'going green', you have a solution that seems to be showing a majority of people in America are letting go of the pharmaceutical-only direction and fusing it with a healthier integrative attitude. These are all your customer/patient base and they will go to the pharmacy that accommodates their health direction. You need to be that pharmacy.

Some interesting information that reinforces your choice includes the fact that Americans continue to buy supplements, even during a questionable economy. A Council for Responsible Nutrition survey indicated 71% (over 2/3) are buying dietary supplements, no matter what the economic trend. Another study by the Council for Responsible Nutrition resulted in finding that those individuals that take dietary supplements make healthier life choices (73%). A Pharmavite survey showed that 1 in 5 consumers are asking their pharmacists questions about vitamins and supplements, as opposed to 1-in-3 consumer questions about OTC.

So, ok, you are sold on the concept of adding an integrative approach; what do you do now? There are a number of layers that you need to look at first to make the right decision. I know, you are now thinking 'I don't have time', but, don't view this as a daunting task or project. This is actually easy, if you take it one step at a time.

1st: Look around in your community to view what other companies are embracing a healthier approach. You may notice that grocery stores have added healthier food offerings, including organic selections and many of the chains and big box pharmacies are including wellness clinics.

2nd: Adding a good, high quality selection of vitamins and supplements in a variety of price levels is key. The good news is, these products offer higher margins and you have the opportunity to increase your pharmacy income to offset any losses from the script side as well as investment to the integrative choice. You may want to work with an integrative consultation service for advisement, but you will also need to partner with some of your local nutritionists and practitioners that are involved in the wellness side.

3rd: You need to differentiate yourself so that your pharmacy has a unique combination for the integrative patient. Changing the pattern of your customers from filling their prescriptions with you and buying supplements elsewhere is part of the task. Getting the 'word out' will involve ensuring that you have in-store signage to catch their attention, but also other marketing arenas, such as a wellness 'web presence'. Marketing is the highest priority, so your website should include the easy, time efficient 'tools' such as: enewsletters, e-coupons, auto selection Facebook feeds, events calendars, email blast abilities and even the opportunity to display your integrative selections on your site. An important factor is that you need to have personal control of your site, so that you can make ad-hoc changes whenever you want. Do not try a 'DIY' or cheaper direction on this. Today's website is the sole view of your pharmacy and if you don't work with a professional integrative web company, your efforts may be stalled or broken. Your website is a direct reflection of you and this must be done right.

4th: As you move forward, the relationships that you have developed with other wellness companies in your community will bring new customers to you. A coordinated marketing effort can include ideas such as mutual flyers and advertising as well as listing on your website as a referral. You can work with your partners to establish special in-pharmacy events, such as nutritional counseling (of special interest to those patients that are overweight or suffer from diabetes).

Since we talk to independent pharmacies across the country, we also know that there seems to be a common theme: independents have a tendency to embrace changing technologies more slowly; independents seem to look at the investment of dollars rather than the larger picture; independents continue to state they don't have the time to make any changes. All of these factors can be game-changers. As humans, we invest in many things that we have to have, but we also spend on things that we want. To make a transition to integrative you need to adopt to take advantage of the fact that you can make changes so much faster than the chains (it takes them months, or even years), work with professional companies that will create an easy-to-use marketing world for you and make that dollar spend with a positive attitude, because there is a good return on investment for you in your future in choosing the integrative approach.

How To Test For Metabolic Syndrome From the Pharmacy

As a pharmacist, you can provide a tremendous benefit in the optimal testing of risk factors for metabolic syndrome.

Although there is no agreed upon official definition of Metabolic syndrome, there is a consensus between the International Diabetes Foundation and the American Heart Association/National Heart, Lung, and Blood Institute which defines Metabolic Syndrome as the presence of any three of the following:

- Increased waist circumference (≥102 cm in men and ≥88 cm in women)
- Elevated blood pressure (≥130/85 mmHg)
- Elevated blood sugar (fasting glucose ≥100 mg/dL)
- Elevated low high-density lipoprotein (>100 mg/dL)
- (HDL) cholesterol (<40 mg/dL in men and <50 mg/dL in women)
- High triglycerides (≥150 mg/dL).

Insulin resistance is often the spark that lights the fire to metabolic syndrome, spurred by diet and lifestyle, although fortunately by addressing issues in a preventative fashion, much can be done for the individual's health.

The closest many people get to addressing testing measures related to insulin resistance and metabolic syndrome are the standard Fasting blood glucose, Hemoglobin A1c, Total Cholesterol, High Blood Pressure, LDL Cholesterol, HDL Cholesterol, Fasting Triglycerides, and at times their own blood glucose testing machine at home.

Where HbA1c has been an advancement providing a history of someone's blood sugar levels, and the other tests certainly have their value, let's take a look at some other tests addressing risk factors often overlooked by the conventional testing schedule above.

Where there are increasing tests based on the continued advanced sciences, these are tests local providers can easily order, and even pharmacists through specialty sa-

Marketing Tip #23- Repurposing

Repurposing is the single best way to leverage your time, your productivity, and your marketing message. It's like a wheel; your message is the hub, **the spokes are your many different channels of media and marketing**, the rim is your customers.

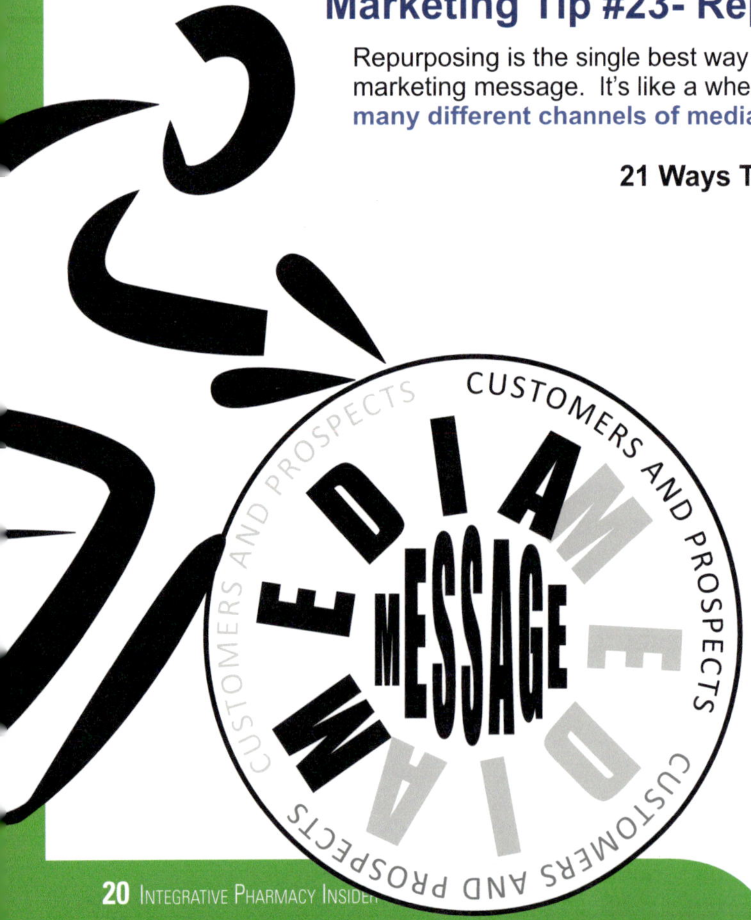

21 Ways To Repurpose checklist:

- ✓ Blog Posts
- ✓ Bag Stuffers
- ✓ Email
- ✓ Print Article's
- ✓ Podcast/Online Audio
- ✓ Video
- ✓ Dr. Marketing
- ✓ Audio CD
- ✓ Paper Transcript
- ✓ Shipping Cards/Ride-alongs
- ✓ Direct Mail
- ✓ PDF Report/Consumer Awareness Guide
- ✓ Newsletters
- ✓ Counter Cards/ Information Sheets
- ✓ Live Workshops
- ✓ Video CD
- ✓ Press Releases
- ✓ Social Media Posts
- ✓ Faxes
- ✓ Book/ebook
- ✓ Door Hangers

Just think, by adding just one new message and one new channel of marketing every month (or week), your marketing efforts will compound exponentially.

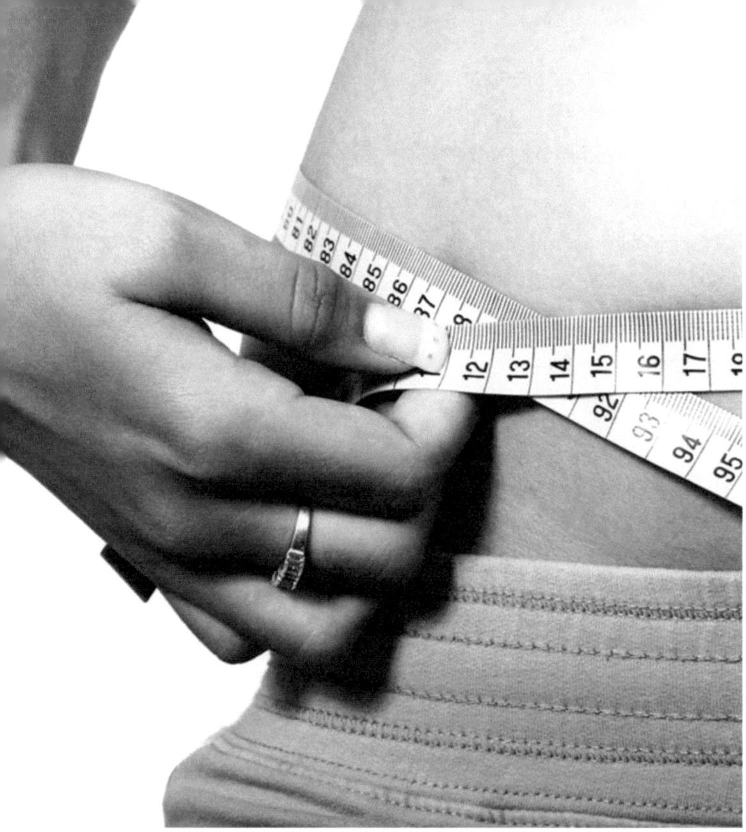

liva and blood spot testing companies, certainly providing a more in depth discussion on ones metabolic profile.

Hemoglobin A1c (HbA1c) – Testing HbA1c provides the average blood sugar level over the past three months, including both fasting and post prandial levels. Due to the fact that blood sugar levels can vary considerably from day to day, HbA1c levels are considered to be a more reliable assessment of one's blood sugar status. A consistent elevation of HbA1c levels can be indicative of loss of blood sugar control, a risk factor of diabetes.

Fasting Insulin – Checking fasting insulin levels is a reliable way of measuring the degree of insulin resistance. Insulin is a hormone produced by the pancreas used by liver, adipose and muscle cells to take up glucose from the blood to immediately convert to energy, or be stored as glycogen in the liver for future use. Insulin resistance usually results in rising insulin levels, often associated with increasing body fat, although can also occur in individuals of normal weight. Insulin resistance can further influence high blood sugar levels and other metabolic disturbances such as altered blood lipid profiles and high blood pressure.

Leptin – Leptin is a hormone which exists primarily in subcutaneous fat which plays a key role in regulating neuroendocrine and immune function, appetite, metabolic rate and body weight. When leptin levels are within healthy limits, it alerts the brain and other body tissues that you have eaten enough and stored away enough fat, and it's now time to burn off some excess fat. When leptin resistance ensues there is interference with leptin signaling often leading to risk factors of metabolic syndrome including high BMI, abdominal obesity, hyperinsulinemia, high triglycerides, low HDL, and inflammation.

Fasting Triglycerides – Triglycerides are the form that fat takes when it is being stored for energy in your body. Triglycerides, liked cholesterol, are vital for human life but unhealthy if at too high a level and can lead to arterial plaque buildup, and often linked with blood sugar dysfunction. High fasting triglycerides levels are another important indicator of atherogenic dyslipidemia and component of metabolic syndrome.

Total Cholesterol, LDL Cholesterol, HDL Cholesterol, and VLDL Cholesterol – A standard cholesterol profile usually consists of measuring Total Cholesterol, LDL Cholesterol and HDL Cholesterol. High levels of total cholesterol, LDL cholesterol and low levels of HDL have consistently been associated with risk of cardiovascular disease and metabolic syndrome. VLDL (Very-low-density lipoprotein) cholesterol is a type of lipoprotein which contains the highest amount of triglyceride. Because it contains a high level of triglyceride, having a high VLDL level means you may have an increased risk of coronary artery disease, which can lead to a heart attack or stroke. Higher amounts and large VLDL particles are also associated with an increased risk of high blood pressure and stroke.

Lipoprotein(A) is a small cholesterol particle that can cause inflammation and clog blood vessels when present in the body in elevated levels. High Lipoprotein A levels can greatly increase a person's risk of developing heart disease. An interesting point is that taking statin drugs to lower your HDL and LDL can actually lead to an increase of Lipoprotein A in the body...thus the critical need for adequate cholesterol and cardiovascular management.

C-Reactive Protein (CRP) - This is a protein produced in the liver and found in the blood which is one of the key indicators of inflammation in the body. C-reactive protein levels become elevated in the presence of an infection or inflammation. CRP levels can also rise due to a previous infections, obesity, and even depression. However a CRP high sensitivity assay (hs-CRP) detects the smaller rises in CRP levels that are associated with metabolic syndrome, thus can be an early indicator of cardiovascular disease and atherosclerosis.

So as we move away from a disease state management health care system to one of a preventative nature, you see that there are many options for which you can play a role in assessment, identification and utilization of natural therapies with your clients.

5 UN-Creative Thoughts About Creativity

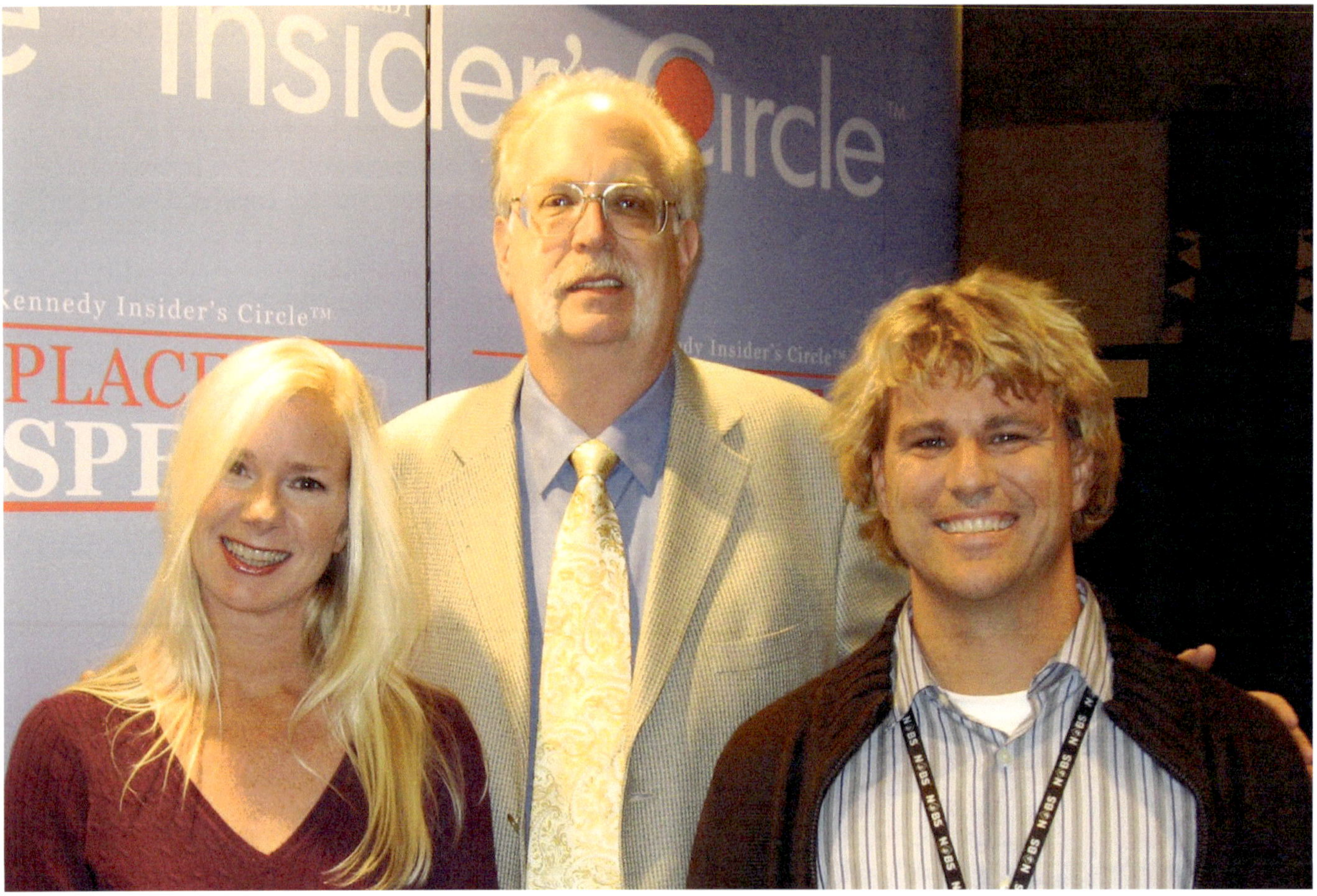

Entrepreneurs and marketers are constantly challenged to be creative. But creativity as it is commonly thought of and practiced is sin not virtue, because it is slow and ponderous; because it begins with a blank slate. One of the most profitably creative entrepreneurs of all time, Walt Disney, said "....stop talking and begin doing." To be profitable in the real world, creativity must be fast, decisive, practical, implementable and implemented. There's little room for creativity for creativity's sake.

I tend to practice "creativity cheating" – and thought I'd give you a few quick "cheats", from the many I talked about at my one day Creative Thinking For Entrepreneurs Seminar.*

#1: STEAL AND ADAPT WHAT'S ALREADY BUILT

From Tony Baxter, Senior V.P., Creative Development/ Imagineering at Disney: "For the climactic scene in the

Indiana Jones Adventure at Disneyland, we wanted the ride vehicle to suddenly start backing up as the giant rolling boulder comes thundering toward us. Having a ride vehicle back up in the middle of a ride is SOMETHING THAT'S NEVER BEEN DONE, BECAUSE IT'S NOT POSSIBLE. With eighteen vehicles traveling down the same track at the same time, a vehicle going in reverse would collide with the next vehicle coming behind it along the track. But if you've ever ridden in the Indiana Jones attraction, you know your vehicle *does* suddenly start backing up. At least that's your perception. Your vehicle has actually stopped. It's the walls and ceiling that are moving, giving you the undeniable feeling that you're traveling backward.......so, where did we come up with this solution? A car wash. One of those self-service machines at the gas station where you pull your car in and park while a series of brushes and spray heads mounted above and beside your car travel back and forth."

There's more to Tony's story, but enough here to make the point: whatever you're trying to do, *somebody* has already figured out and built --- just not in your business or industry or in an application you might ordinarily, easily think of in connection with your business. You do NOT want to invest umpteen days, weeks, months duplicating all the figuring out and innovation and engineering – you want to find the thing that's already built.

Oh, and a key question to ask every time you see anything, go anywhere, experience anything: *how can I use that?*

#2: WORK BACKWARDS

Most people approach creative thinking from the front – the idea. Let's say you're going to open up a new restaurant. You'll probably start with the name, maybe the theme, the menu. But the best place to start is with what will insure a customer keeps coming back. Or his final few minutes in the place. What goes on at the cash register. What will create the highest average ticket. In short, you start thinking about outcomes and then build backwards. Right now, in the movie business, a ton of very important money comes from stealth advertising and product placement. So very, very, very early in the creative process, in many cases prior to script and definitely prior to picking actors, the list of every possible product/advertiser that can be integrated into the film is thought through. I am told in one blockbuster movie of 2005, a scene that took place inside a ski resort's dim-lit bar at night in the book was moved to daytime, outside on the restaurant's deck because they could get a sunglasses company, a parka company, and a liquor company with its name on patio table umbrellas to pony up money.

#3: BE MARKET / BUYER DRIVEN IN (ALMOST) EVERYTHING YOU DO

I started out, ever so briefly, in the 'traditional' advertising business, and have occasionally been involved – such as a few years back when I butted heads with Weight Watchers' big name Madison Avenue agency. They tend to start their creative process with random ideas. If you watch the advertising-related exercises on 'The Apprentice', you've seen this same mistake made. So, gather a bunch of ad industry creative types together to talk about advertising for a new perfume, they'll instantly leap off a dozen creative cliffs: names, colors, package, celebrity, music. I say: wait a damn minute! Tell me who the 'target' is – don't even bother telling me about the product. I don't give a rat's patootie that it smells like jasmine or ocean breezes or beached whales in the last throes of death or is made from cedar planks or horny minks' glandular secretions. I want to work backwards from who the intended buyer is. And it matters whether she's 18, 25, 30, 35, 40, 45, 50, 55, single, married, etc. I catch clients constantly playing BLIND ARCHERY. Don't develop a product or service or offer or Marketing Message unless you are developing it *for* a particular somebody. Not only is that the best and surest way to make money and avoid flops, it's a terrific creativity shortcut because it narrows your range of creative work from the git-go. If you want to manage time better, by now you probably know my best strategy is to give yourself less loose time to manage. If you want to get through the creation process quicker, give yourself a smaller canvass.

#4: SWIPE, SWIPE, SWIPE, SWIPE (LEGALLY & ETHICALLY)

I get real joy out of hearing from GKIC Members as I did the day I wrote this, and hearing one after another telling me how they took an example from the *NO B.S. MARKETING LETTER,* etc., etc. Again, you should never start with a blank slate. Too hard, too slow. Gather up some stuff to give you a jump start.

#5: DOODADS AS INSPIRATION

One of my favorite shortcuts is finding the little doodads, promotional items, grabbers that are available, that suggest or furnish the theme for my marketing campaign --- especially when doing direct-mail. The copywriting I did for Rory Fatt's boot camp one year, 'The Magical Business Life Boot Camp For Restaurant Owners', was because I first found a bunch of magic stuff in the Oriental Trading catalogs: tricks, cards, top hats, etc. I picked the theme because these things were available cheap.

If you don't get these catalogs, you must:

Hands On Fun – Creative Tools
www.handsonfun.com

Oriental Trading/Business
www.orientaltrading.com

Fun Impressions
www.funimpressions.com

Here are just a few items that beget ideas:

Magnetic Construction Set

"Build a better _____________"

Foam Fall Leaves

"The leaves have started to turn colors – your reminder to __________"

Dinosaurs

"Once upon a time, mighty dinosaurs ruled the earth. They no longer even exist/ Why? Because they didn't adapt to change. Don't risk extinction!"

Jumbo Foam Dice

'If you want to gamble, go to Vegas.

If you want a sure thing: ________________"

Seasonal Themes....a little more obvious.

For example, Chinese New Years, St. Patricks Day

So, for example, instead of the Magic theme, next year Rory might use : Build A Better Restaurant Business. There's the construction set I just talked about, hard hats, toy hammers and tool kits, sales letters printed on architects' blueprints, building permits, and on and on and on. Who else could use this? Kitchen remodelers.....fitness center (build a better body)......karate school (build a better kid)....

See, wandering through one of these catalogs is another creativity shortcut.

There's a business term: "speed to market." It's extremely important. The entrepreneurs I work with who make the most money are "speed to market" people. They rely on creativity shortcuts. You should too.

DAN S. KENNEDY is a serial, multi-millionaire entrepreneur; highly paid and sought after marketing and business strategist; advisor to countless first-generation, from-scratch multi-millionaire and 7-figure income entrepreneurs and professionals; and, in his personal practice, one of the very highest paid direct-response copywriters in America. As a speaker, he has delivered over 2,000 compensated presentations, appearing repeatedly on programs with the likes of Donald Trump, Gene Simmons (KISS), Debbi Fields (Mrs. Fields Cookies), and many other celebrity-entrepreneurs, for former U.S. Presidents and other world leaders, and other leading business speakers like Zig Ziglar, Brian Tracy and Tom Hopkins, often addressing audiences of 1,000 to 10,000 and up. His popular books have been favorably recognized by Forbes, Business Week, Inc. and Entrepreneur Magazine. His NO B.S. MARKETING LETTER, one of the business newsletters published for Members of Glazer-Kennedy Insider's Circle, is the largest paid subscription newsletter in its genre in the world. **Click Here To Claim Your $633.91 Worth of Pure, Powerful, Money-Making Information...For Free**

Home from the Hill
Compounders on Capitol Hill 2012!

More than 300 community pharmacists and pharmacy technicians from across the United States traveled to Washington, D.C., to meet with their federal House and Senate delegations as part of the International Academy of Compounding Pharmacists (IACP) **2012 *Compounders on Capitol Hill* 18th annual conference and legislative event** held, June 23-26, 2012.

In addition to talking to Congress about the importance of having access to personalized medicines, IACP Members specifically addressed the importance of complete Medicare, Medicaid and other prescription insurance coverage for all compounded preparations.

"IACP is continuing to educate patients, prescribers, pharmacists, patient advocacy groups, congressional offices, state pharmacy associations, state pharmacy boards and Medicaid divisions about the vital importance of continued access to compounded medications. These visits to Congress came at a particularly critical time for compounding pharmacies across the country and for the patients whom they serve. Every pharmacist, pharmacist technician and prescriber who joined us on Capitol Hill this year and those patients and prescribers who have called and written their members of Congress were vital to ensuring that our voices continue to be heard," says **IACP Executive Vice President & CEO David G. Miller, RPh.**

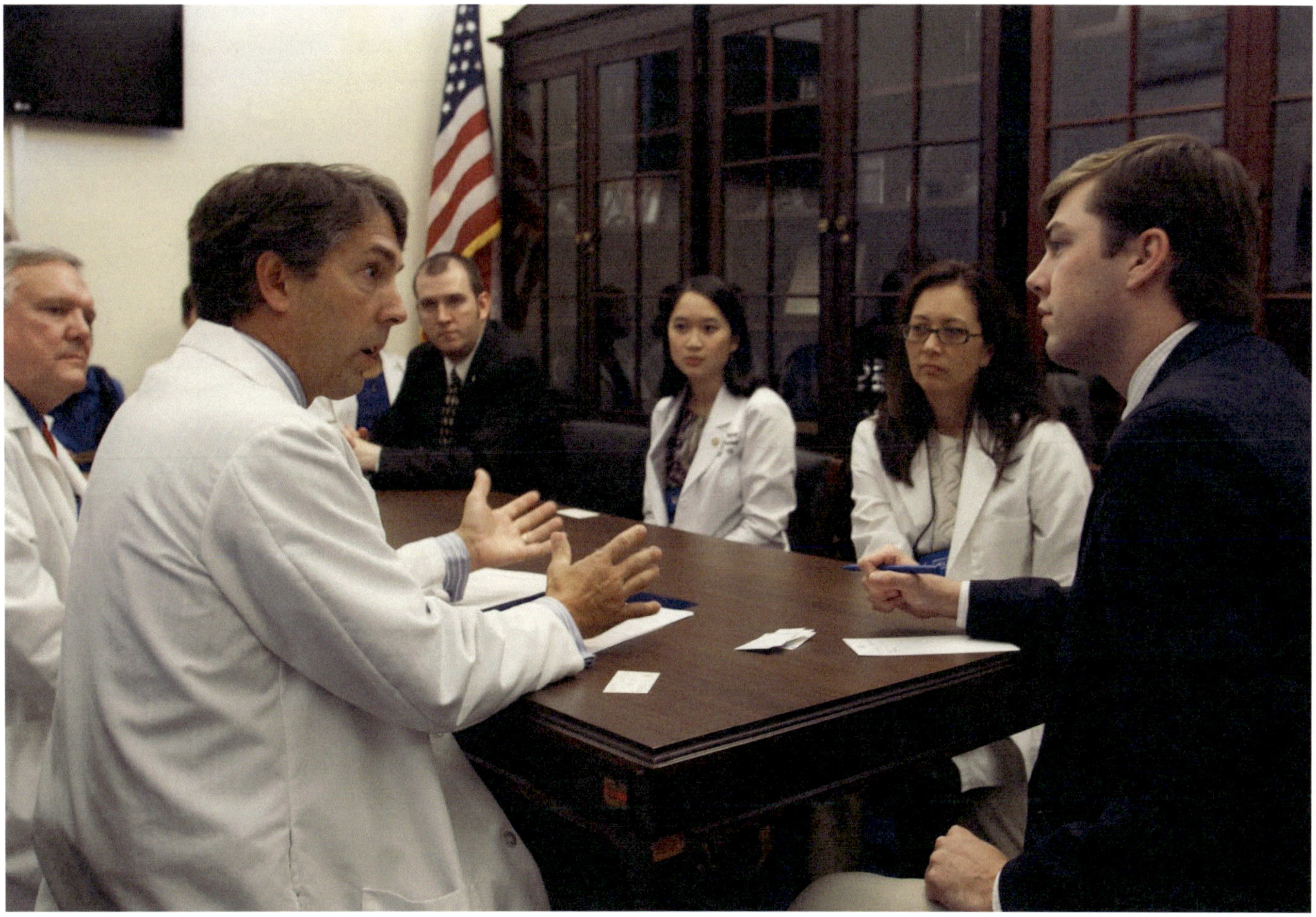

The CCH 2012 Asks:

Constructive Transfer - Request formal rule-making by the Drug Enforcement Administration on constructive transfer

Request fair and equitable treatment of all pharmacy providers by the Centers for Medicare & Medicaid Services (CMS)

Request consistent policy on coverage of compounded preparations under CMS programs (Medicaid/Medicare)

CCH in Action: Congressional Letters Sent to DEA on Constructive Transfer

The IACP Team hit the ground running after wrapping up another successful *Compounders on Capitol Hill* (CCH)! One of the primary CCH 2012 Asks involved a formal rule-making request issued to the Drug Enforcement Administration (DEA) on constructive transfer of controlled substances. Letters to the DEA on this key patient issue were sent from both the House and Senate to the agency at the end of July.

IACP Members who attended this year's *Compounders on Capitol Hill* (CCH) played a vital role in lobbying their respective Members of Congress, asking them to support either the House or Senate letter.

The House letter, championed by Congressman Ted Poe (R-TX), and the Senate letter championed by Senator John Cornyn (R-TX), quickly enlisted the support of several key congressional members due in large part to the groundwork done by pharmacists attending CCH 2012.

Please visit IACP's website at www.iacprx.org for a complete listing of all congressional support and current status for this effort.

Your Participation at Compounders on Capitol Hill is Vital!

IACP's mission for CCH 2013 is to encourage even more participation at the actual Hill Day event held during CCH. Hill Day is one of the most important CCH events and will bring your D.C. experience full circle. Plan to stay through Hill Day next year so that you can ensure the IACP Asks are being communicated to your state's representatives. States without CCH attendees this year included: Alaska, District of Columbia, Hawaii, Idaho, Maine, Maryland, Montana, Nevada, New Hampshire, Rhode Island, Vermont, West Virginia, and Wyoming. *We look forward to having your colleagues' representation in these states next year!*

Hill Day 2012 Stats at a Glance

IACP once again worked with Soapbox Consulting, LLC, a D.C.-based consultant specializing in grass-roots advocacy. Soapbox's **Christopher Kush** shared insider tips with CCH participants on how to ensure an effective congressional office visit as well as insider tips on how to not only "get your voices heard, but your messages remembered!" IACP's **Executive Vice President & CEO David G. Miller, RPh**, and **Vice President of Government Affairs Sarah Dodge** conducted a "Being a Good Advocate for Compounding" session. This interactive session provided techniques to successfully convey our position and message to legislators.

126 total participants representing 37 states

183 face-to-face meetings scheduled

74% of Senate offices scheduled

24.71% of House offices scheduled

42 meetings included the Senator/Congressman

Please Note: These stats do not include the additional "drop-in" congressional office visits that took place as opportunities presented themselves!

Save the Date – CCH 2013!

The 19th Annual *Compounders on Capitol Hill* will take place at the Crystal City Gateway Marriott in 2013. Stay tuned for more excited details to come! Many improvements are already in the works based on your suggestions and feedback.

19th Annual *Compounders on Capitol Hill*
June 1-4, 2013
Crystal City Gateway Marriott
Arlington, VA

Integrative Pharmacy Success Example

If It Works For Your Colleagues, It Can Work For You

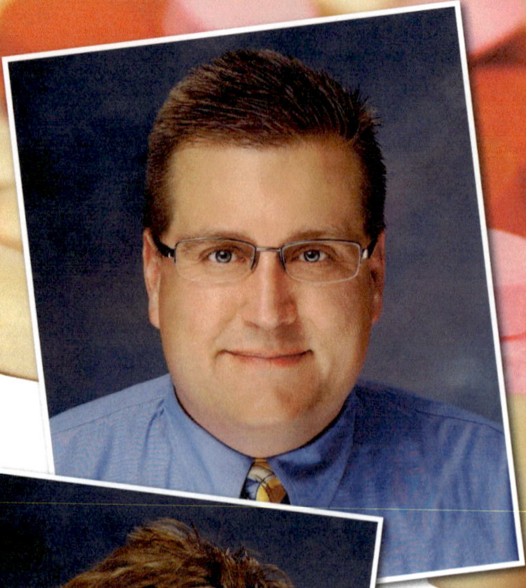

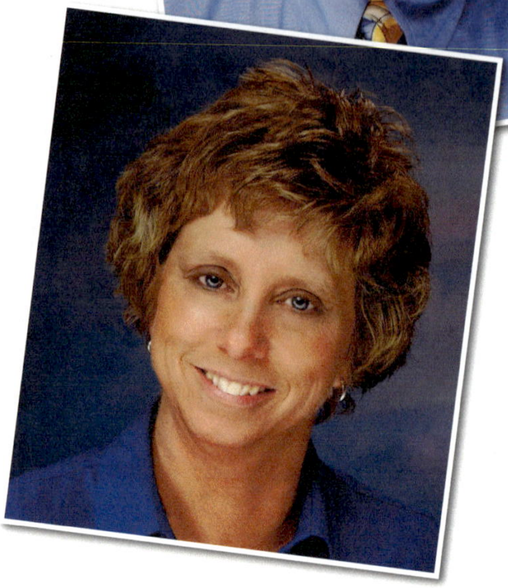

In this issue for the Integrative Pharmacy Success Example, we shine the light on Wade Siefert RPh and Jennifer Siefert, RPh - Owners of Preckshot Professional Pharmacy in Peoria Heights, Illinois. Preckshot Professional Pharmacy is a compounding-only pharmacy which continually emulates what an independent pharmacy can be.

After speaking to Wade and Jennifer, I felt it was important to share a couple of strategies which they are implementing at Preckshot, that work really well to sell more wellness - strategies which everyone can and should be doing.

Q. Wade and Jen, first off, can you give us an idea of the breakdown of your business, what products and services you offer?

A. In our Practice we are currently tallying sales at 23% Nutritional Supplements and 77% Compounding.

Q. So it is apparent that nutrition, integrative and lifestyle medicine are a growing part of your practice. We often coach people on the fact that it's not that difficult, expensive or time consuming to market and communicate with your current customers (the easiest and least expensive people to market to) to sell more wellness. You mentioned a new strategy that you have implemented at your Pharmacy which is working really well to sell more nutrition. Would you mind sharing that with us?

A. We work closely with our Master Marketer Nicholas Maloof, Project Specialist Kayla Livingston, and Compounding Pharmacy Marketing Partner and Web Master Patti Storey in the 'full spectrum marketing' of our "Preckshot Personal Vitamin of the Month" promotion. We take the designated Vitamin of that month and we cross-market it through a huge arsenal of "branded" media such as:

- Preckshot Pipeline Info Sheets / Faxes and Counter Cards
- Preckshot Bag Stuffers
- Preckshot Enclosure Cards accompany all of our shipped orders
- Place in select Preckshot Print Newspaper ads
- Broadcasting each month's Vitamin of the Month on our Preckshot Personal Radio Program's 'Nutrition in the News Segment.'
- Highlighting the Vitamin of the month in our Preckshot Pages Magazines
- Through our Preckshot Social Media Network of Facebook, Constant Contact, Pinterest and soon to be launched Preckshot You Tube Channel for the world to enjoy

- Preckshot In-Store Displays and Reading Materials noting specifically the extra discount applicable to that Vitamin/Supplement of the Month.
- Our Preckshot Point Of Sale System can also send e-mails to customers who have previously purchased these items to alert them about the current month's Preckshot Personal Promotion.

Q- That's awesome, and one thing that stands out is the constant branding of "Preckshot", there is no way someone can get through this article without knowing what pharmacy we are talking about.

I think people often overlook some simple tools that they are using on a daily basis - things that can alternatively be used for other reasons than their main intention, such as your Preckshot point of sale system in the example above. You mentioned another monthly marketing strategy which utilizes your POS as well, which does not take much time and is highly effective for selling more supplements: Can you share this with us?

A- We flag our Preckshot Patient's birthdays in our POS System. We then print those files by the month and mail our Customers a Preckshot Praise Birthday Card (custom photo of our staff) and a 25% off coupon to be used within a designated period of time. The coupon is for OTC's only and pays big dividends in generating additional and ongoing Vitamin and Nutritional Supplement sales

In Summary:

I like the fact that you are using your POS System. Many people's knee-jerk reaction might be to go to their pharmacy patient system and download files. The fact is, we might have some customers who are not prescription clients, but are exclusively OTC Customers. Ignoring this demographic could prove to be a huge missed opportunity for many.

It is apparent that anyone can do any of these examples, even if all staff members are not well versed in nutrition. With the help of the pharmacist, they can have an easy, cost-effective and consistent marketing stream, which promotes continued nutritional sales.

What I find often stands in the way of pharmacists growing their nutritional business as they should, is lack of implementation. Things just do not get done. These examples by Wade and Jennifer Siefert and the Preckshot Professional Pharmacy Staff, in conjunction with their Master Marketer and Colleagues, show how the challenges of cost, time or expertise have no bearing on success. It's about initiative... and if you're serious about success... a 'full spectrum' marketing effort like the one "implemented" at Preckshot Professional Pharmacy.

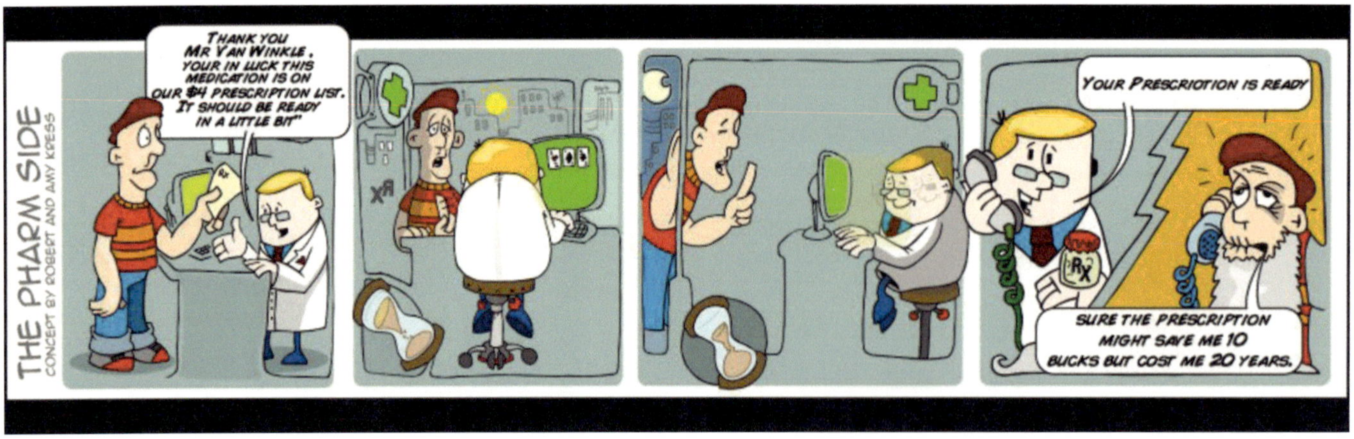

Nutritional Support For Metabolic Syndrome With Berberine

Robert B Kress, RPh
Clinical pharmacist, founder and publisher of Pharmacist Integrative

TARGET AUDIENCE:

This accredited program is targeted to pharmacists, pharmacists technicians, and nurses practicing in hospital and community pharmacies. Estimated time to complete this monograph and post test is 90 minutes.

DISCLAIMER:

PharmCon, Inc does not view the existence of relationships as an implication of bias or that the value of the material is decreased. The content of the activity was planned to be balanced and objective. Occasionally, authors may express opinions that represent their own viewpoint. Participants have an implied responsibility to use the newly acquired information to enhance patient outcomes and their own professional development. The information presented in this activity is not meant to serve as a guideline for patient or pharmacy management. Conclusions drawn by participants should be derived from objective analysis of scientific data presented from this monograph and other unrelated sources.

Program Overview:

To provide pharmacists and nurses with an understanding of Nutritional Support For Metabolic Syndrome With Berberine

OBJECTIVES:

After completing this program, participants will be able to:

1. Explain the impact of metabolic syndrome and the implications on the health care system.
2. Identify the goals of assessment, prevention and treatment of metabolic syndrome.
3. Address downfalls of conventional prescription therapy related to treating metabolic syndrome.
4. Describe roles and benefits of berberine in metabolic syndrome.
5. Provide general nutritional recommendations to patients based on individual or complementary therapy with berberine and other synergistic supplements.

CE for this lesson can be obtained online at

freeCE PharmCon

www.freece.com/integrative

Introduction

In 1988, researchers noted that several risk factors (e.g., dyslipidemia, hypertension, and hyperglycemia) commonly clustered together which he called Syndrome X. Researchers and practitioners have postulated that insulin resistance underlies Syndrome X (hence the commonly used term insulin resistance syndrome). Other researchers use the term metabolic syndrome for this clustering of metabolic risk factors, which avoids the implication that insulin resistance is the only cause of associated risk factors, although as you will see it plays a very big role.

Where cardiovascular disease (CVD) has been identified as the primary clinical outcome of the metabolic syndrome, most people with metabolic syndrome have insulin resistance which confers an increased risk for type 2 diabetes. When diabetes becomes clinically apparent, CVD risk rises sharply.

Beyond CVD and type 2 diabetes, metabolic syndrome has been implicated in driving almost every chronic disease and individuals with metabolic syndrome seemingly are susceptible to other conditions including; heart attacks, stroke, depression, arthritis, dementia, Alzheimer's disease, polycystic ovary syndrome (PCOS), infertility, fatty liver, cholesterol gallstones, asthma, sleep disturbances, obesity and some forms of cancer.

Although there is no agreed upon official definition of metabolic syndrome, there is a consensus between the International Diabetes Foundation and the American Heart Association/National Heart, Lung, and Blood Institute which defines metabolic syndrome as the presence of any three of the following:

- Increased waist circumference (≥102 cm in men and ≥88 cm in women)
- Elevated blood pressure (≥130/85 mmHg)
- Elevated blood sugar (fasting glucose ≥100 mg/dL)
- Elevated low high-density lipoprotein (>100 mg/dL)
- (HDL) cholesterol (<40 mg/dL in men and <50 mg/dL in women)
- High triglycerides (≥150 mg/dL).

Alzheimer's disease is now being linked to metabolic syndrome and insulin resistance in what is being called Type 3 Diabetes, also referred to as Brain Diabetes. This dangerous hybrid form of Diabetes was confirmed during a study which took place at Brown University's Medical School. That study showed for the first time exactly how the brain produces and uses insulin, which very closely mirrors the way that the pancreas makes it.

The problem with Type 3 Diabetes is Protein Plaque. The way the brain makes insulin can result in the formation of this plaque, which resembles that which is found in Diabetes Type 1 and Diabetes Type 2 sufferers. However, the attack of the brain's functions is the result with Type 3

Diabetes, and memory loss and improper memory creation and formation are the result.

Now that it is established that much of the growing rates of metabolic syndrome are due to the rising rates of insulin resistance, pre-diabetes and diabetes, thus leading to a host of other disease states, the statistics related to states of health, as well as the financial burden upon a health care system, are startling:

- Type 1 diabetes rose 23% among young people during the first nine years of the 21st century, while type 2 increased by 21%.
- One in two Americans are now pre-diabetic or diabetic.
- In 1990, there was not a single state in the country where obesity was over 20%.
- In 2012, there is not a single state in the country where the obesity rate is under 20%.
- Almost 70% of Americans are overweight.
- It is estimated that in 20 years ½ Americans will be clinically obese.
- About $174 billion was spent to treat diabetes in the U.S. last year, while chronic diseases in total accounted for about 75% of total healthcare spending.
- Some models forecast the number of affected people doubling to between 50 million and 55 million by 2025 from 26 million in the U.S. today.
- The diabetes nutritional supplement category has seen explosive growth, sales increasing 50% over the last four years, and forecasts show it will continue to grow at an explosive pace.

Diet and Lifestyle

Where we have established that insulin resistance is often the spark that ignites the fires of metabolic syndrome, the majority of cases can be avoided and prevented by diet and lifestyle measures alone. This brings upon a need for the role of a practitioner to be an advocate for measures of diet and lifestyle, as well as addressing the upstream cause instead of just waiting to treat the downstream problem. One does not have to be an expert in this area, and there are some simple dietary and lifestyle recommendations which have proven to be successful in decreasing risk factors of insulin resistance and metabolic syndrome. They are as follows:

- Promoting regular physical activities appropriate for the individual's state of health.

- Eating wholefoods, avoiding preservatives, artificial colors and artificial flavorings in foods.
- Eliminate refined sugars and carbohydrates from diet.
- Reduce or eliminate liquid calories.
- Eating small meals throughout the day, every 3 to 4 hours with a protein at each meal.
- Understand the importance of healthy fats in one's diet.
- Understand the importance of not skipping breakfast.

Testing and Assessment:

Given the risk factors for Metabolic Syndrome it is quite easy to assess, test and track a client's health, which allows one to take a proactive approach with lifestyle adjustments such as diet and possibly nutritional supplementation support.

Below you will find the tests which can be done by the patient's primary caregiver while pharmacists can provide such services in expanding their clinical based roles through in house testing and specialty saliva and blood spot testing companies.

Hemoglobin A1c (HbA1c) – Testing HbA1c provides the average blood sugar level over the past three months, including both fasting and post prandial levels. Due to the fact that blood sugar levels can vary considerably from day to day, HbA1c levels are considered to be a more reliable assessment to track one's blood sugar status. A consistent elevation of HbA1c levels can be indicative of loss of blood sugar control, a risk factor of diabetes.

Fasting Insulin – Checking fasting insulin levels is a reliable way of measuring the degree of insulin resistance. Insulin is a hormone produced by the pancreas that is used by liver, adipose and muscle cells to take up glucose from the blood to immediately convert to energy, or be stored as glycogen in the liver for future use. Insulin resistance usually results in rising insulin levels, often associated with increasing body fat, although it can also occur in individuals of normal weight. Insulin resistance can further influence high blood sugar levels and other metabolic disturbances such as altered blood lipid profiles and high blood pressure.

Fasting Triglycerides – Triglycerides are the form that fat takes when it is being stored for energy in your body. Triglycerides, liked cholesterol, are vital for human life but unhealthy if at too high a level and can lead to arterial plaque buildup, and often linked with blood sugar dysfunction. High fasting triglycerides levels are another important indicator of atherogenic dyslipidemia and a component of metabolic syndrome.

Total Cholesterol, LDL Cholesterol, HDL Cholesterol, and VLDL Cholesterol – A standard cholesterol profile usually consists of measuring Total Cholesterol, LDL Cholesterol and HDL Cholesterol. High levels of total cholesterol, LDL cholesterol and low levels of HDL have consistently been associated with risk of cardiovascular disease and metabolic syndrome. VLDL (Very-low-density lipoprotein) cholesterol is a type of lipoprotein which contains the highest amount of triglyceride. Because it contains a high level of triglyceride, having a high VLDL level means you may have an increased risk of coronary artery disease, which can lead to a heart attack or stroke. Higher amounts and large VLDL particles are also associated with an increased risk of high blood pressure and stroke.

Blood Pressure - Hypertension, or high blood pressure, is a key symptom of Metabolic Syndrome. Both conditions are important risk factors in developing Cardiovascular Disease, which can lead to a heart attack or stroke. If left untreated, hypertension can also lead to a wide variety of other life-threatening conditions, such as kidney damage and congestive heart failure. Several studies have proven that Insulin Resistance and the resulting hyperinsulinemia (elevated insulin in the blood) cause increases in blood pressure. This is because elevated levels of insulin can cause atherosclerosis, which directly affects the diameter of the inside of the blood vessel.

Common Prescription Drug Therapies for Metabolic Disorders:

Given the number of disease state risk factors related to metabolic syndrome, there are numerous prescription drugs prescribed. It is important to realize that the goal of prescription therapy is help reduces someone's risk factors; it is often not without side-effects or other challenges. Below are some of the common drug therapies, as well as issues which have in the past or might present themselves, allowing the practitioner to intervene for the good of the patient's health. Here we will be focusing on the two main common risk factors of the metabolic syndrome umbrella based on drug classed prescribed; insulin/blood sugar medications and cholesterol lowering medications.

“I think everyone should use probiotics, and **Dr. Ohhira’s Probiotics®** are the very best brand I have found.”

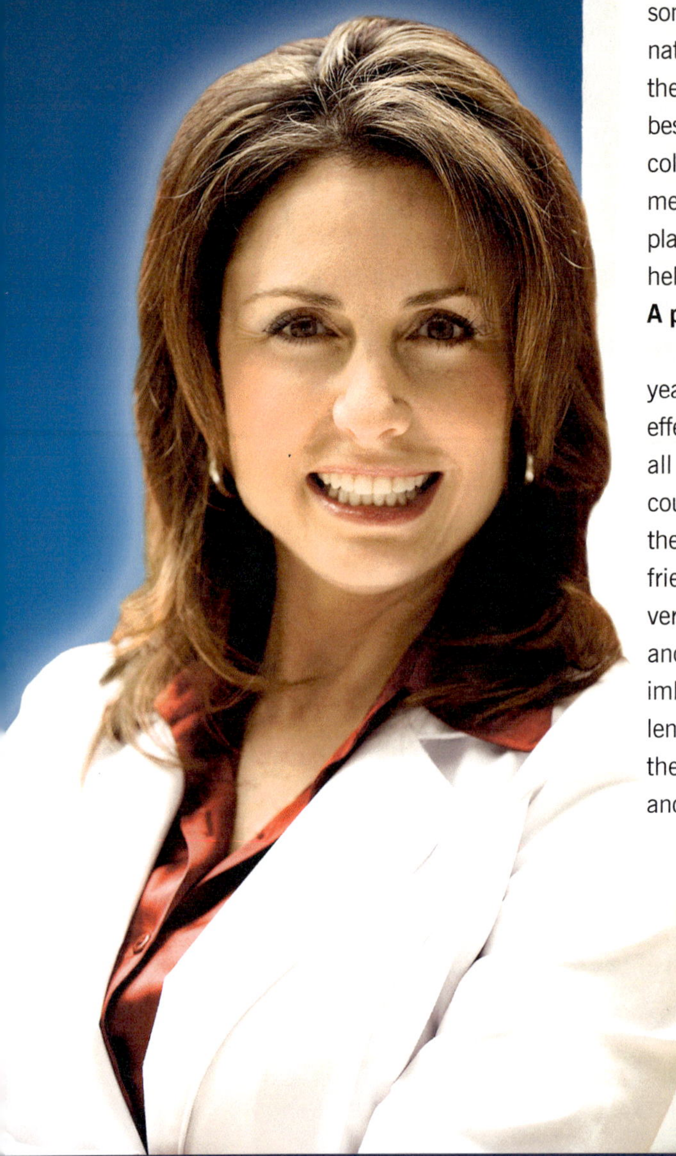

Drug Muggers:

What can you do when a “cure” steals your health?

“America’s Most Trusted Pharmacist” Reveals How Probiotics Support Whole Health Without Side Effects

Prescription and over-the-counter drugs help millions of people with serious health challenges. But in the process, some medications can deplete the body’s natural stores of vitamins and minerals—the very nutrients you need to feel your best. Author, pharmacist, and syndicated columnist, Suzy Cohen refers to certain medications as “drug muggers”. She explains how natural health approaches can help restore whole health.

A personal message from Suzy Cohen:

“In pharmacy school over twenty years ago, I learned about the life-saving effects of many medicines. But virtually all medications, prescribed or over-the-counter, are what I call ‘drug muggers’ – they can affect your body’s population of friendly bacteria. These probiotics are very important; they help you digest food and support immune response. Probiotic imbalance can lead to other health challenges down the line, since every part of the body depends on healthy digestion and an effective immune response.

In my years of experience I have found that Dr. Ohhira’s Probiotics® are the most effective probiotic supplement, and it may be taken in conjunction with prescribed medications. The innovative formula uses twelve strains of carefully selected lactic acid bacteria in a unique Japanese fermentation process. The result is a supplement that encourages the growth of your own unique probiotics.

This synergetic approach is much more effective than simply dumping billions of one bacterial strain into your system, a common approach that can actually trigger an immune response. This distinction sets Dr. Ohhira’s Probiotics® apart from all other brands and makes it my number one recommendation.”

Suzy Cohen, RPh, *has been a licensed pharmacist for more than twenty years and writes the syndicated health column “Dear Pharmacist.” She has been featured on* The View *and* The Dr. Oz Show *and is a member of the Institute of Functional Medicine, American College for Advancement in Medicine, and the American Association of Anti-Aging Medicine.*

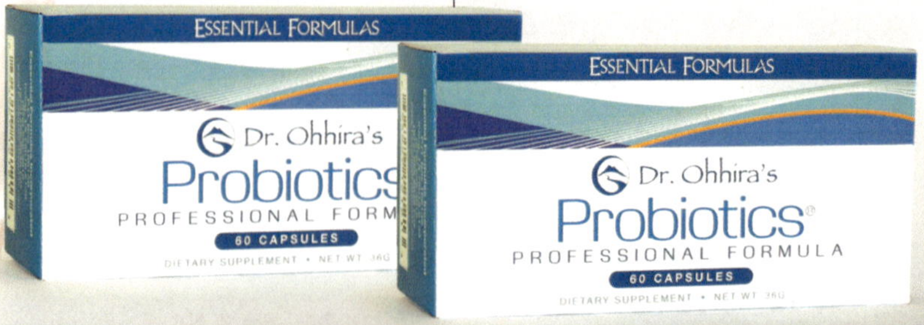

Find Dr. Ohhira’s Probiotics® at fine pharmacies everywhere. No refrigeration necessary.
Visit www.EssentialFormulas.com. Become a friend of Dr. Ohhira on Facebook.

* These statements have not been evaluated by the Food and Drug Administration. This product is not intended to diagnose, treat, cure or prevent any disease.

Diabetes Medications

Metformin

In many cases metformin has become the drug of choice for patients with type II diabetes or rising insulin resistance, although it is important to recognize the increasing prevalence of B12 deficiencies which could mask themselves as diabetic neuropathies.

Metformin (Glucophage ®) is often the first drug of first choice for many conditions of diabetes, whether you are pre-diabetic or have diagnosed diabetes. And by many counts metformin is considered a good drug with a very low side-effect profile, except for the possibility that it can make you B12 deficient, thus resulting in peripheral neuropathies.

This is related to malabsorption of Vitamin B12 due to intrinsic factor deficiency and possibly other mechanisms, in as many as 30% of treated patients.

Researchers presenting at the American Diabetes Association Scientific Sessions summer 2012 noted that:

Chronic metformin use has been previously shown to be associated with vitamin B12 deficiency. Peripheral neuropathy is typically diagnosed as diabetic neuropathy, but this can also be a symptom of vitamin B12 deficiency.

As you can see, this opens up the opportunity for the health care practitioners to identify and address such needs through medication therapy changes and nutritional supplementation.

Thiazolidinediones

Both Avandia® (rosiglitazone) and Actos® (pioglitazone) are in the family of diabetes medications known as thiazolidinediones. They work by increasing an individual's sensitivity to insulin, thus directly combating the insulin resistance. As we have seen in recent years, they do not come without their own downfalls or side- effects.

Rosglitazone

Rosglitazone (Avandia®) has been severely restricted in its prescribing due to a list of cardiac risk events it has shown to be responsible for. One study estimated that from 1999 to 2009, more than 47,000 people taking Avandia needlessly suffered a heart attack, stroke or heart failure, or died.This has led the FDA to restrict the prescribing of rosglitazone United States where patients will be allowed access to the medicine only if they and their doctors attest that they have tried every other diabetes medicine and that patients have been made aware of the drug's substantial risks to the heart. The guidelines continue to warn that because of the risk of serious side effects, rosiglitazone should only be used to treat people who are already taking the medication, or people whose blood sugar cannot be controlled with other medications and who have decided not to take pioglitazone for medical reasons.

In addition to the cardiac events, other side-effects include liver problems, and an increased possibility of breaking of bones, which are all enhanced risk factors and disease states for the diabetic population.

Pioglitazone

Pioglitazone (Actos®) also carries with it a black box warning for congestive heart failure and myocardial infarction and shares other side-effects with rosiglitazone including weight gain, liver problems, increased chance of breaking bones, and something unique to pioglitazone, an increase risk of developing bladder cancer.

Cholesterol Lowering Medications

HMG CoA Reductase Inhibitors - Statins

Since statins are the #1 class of drugs for lowering your cholesterol, we will focus on them. Where statins have shown to be very effective in lowering cholesterol, they too do not come free of side-effects and risks.

First and foremost is their depletion of CoQ10, which is a key nutrient for the mitochondria to create energy, as well as a powerful antioxidant. This is why it is often recommended while taking statins to supplement with a high quality Coenzyme Q10 supplement.

In addition to challenging mitochondrial health which is responsible for healthy aging, statins have also been implicated in a 9% increase in diabetes; thus a patient population under the metabolic syndrome umbrella who have an increased chance of insulin resistance and diabetes, proper prescribing assessment and management of statin drugs is important.

Nutritional Therapy for Metabolic Syndrome- Berberine

Berberine is an alkaloid present in a number of plants, including Berberis vulgaris (European barberry), Berberis aristata (tree turmeric or Indian barberry), Berberis aquifolium (Oregon grape), Hydrastis canadensis (goldenseal), and Coptis chinensis (goldthread). In nutritional practice and therapy, berberine has been most well-known for its antimicrobial activity (against bacteria, viruses, protozoans, helminthes, fungi, and Chlamydia). Over the past few years there has been increasing interest in berberines pleotropic profile, its ability to influence a positive effect on metabolic syndrome including blood-sugar management, lipid lowering, insulin sensitivity, cardiac support, and weight management.

Metabolic Syndrome

Berberine has been shown to help modulate and support many of the risk factors associated with metabolic syndrome.

In a small pilot study of adults (n=7 in final analysis) with a body mass index (BMI) of ≥30, subjects were given 500 mg berberine three times daily for 12 weeks. Several aspects of metabolic syndrome improved, including a 23-percent decrease in triglycerides (from 134.9 mg/dL to 103.4 mg/dL), a 12-percent decrease in total cholesterol (from 197.6 mg/dL to 173.4 mg/dL), and an average weight loss of five pounds (not statistically significant). Where the five pound average weight loss was not statistically significant, it is important to recognize that changes in diet were not performed and the weight loss is believed to be due to berberines' ability to activate AMPK Activated Protein Kinase, another potential mechanism in treating obesity and diabetes.

Thirty-two evaluable hyperlipidemic patients were given 500 mg berberine twice daily for three months, while 11 patients received placebo. Subjects taking berberine experienced a 35-percent reduction in triglycerides, a 29-percent reduction in total cholesterol, and a 25-percent reduction in low-density lipoprotein (LDL) cholesterol (all statistically significant); HDL-cholesterol was unchanged.

In a study of 89 women with polycystic ovary syndrome and associated insulin resistance, berberine significantly decreased waist-to-hip ratio and LDL-cholesterol compared to metformin. Compared to placebo, berberine significantly decreased the area under the curve for insulin, triglycerides, total- and LDL-cholesterol, and increased HDL-cholesterol.

In a three-month clinical study, 116 subjects with type 2 diabetes and dyslipidemia received either 1 g berberine daily or a placebo. Statistically significant decreases were seen in the berberine group in fasting and post-prandial glucose levels, hemoglobin A1c (HbA1c), triglycerides, and total- and LDL-cholesterol.11

In a two-month study, 50 type 2 diabetic patients were assigned to 1 g berberine HCl (500 mg twice daily)and compared to 26 patients on metformin and 21 patients on rosiglitazone.

Similar significant reductions in fasting glucose and HbA1c were seen in both groups, while only the berberine group experienced significant decreases in triglycerides.12 In another three-month study, 36 individuals with newly diagnosed type 2 diabetes were given 500 mg three times daily of berberine or metformin.

Significant improvements in glucose metabolism (fasting and post-prandial glucose and HbA1c) were seen in both groups (e.g., berberine resulted in a decrease of HbA1c from 9.47 +/-0.65 to 7.48 +/- 0.40), while berberine was more effective than metformin at decreasing total cholesterol.13 These same researchers performed a similar study in 48 poorly controlled type 2 diabetics. Berberine (500 mg three times daily), added to their current regimen for three months, resulted in significant decreases from baseline in fasting glucose, postprandial glucose, and HbA1c.

In addition to mechanisms discussed above in terms of its effect on insulin sensitivity, berberine was shown in an animal model to inhibit gluconeogenesis. It also appears to enhance anaerobic glycolysis, producing ATP from glucose, and may even protect pancreatic beta cells from destruction. Other studies have found berberine can prevent the development of advanced glycation end-products and increase production of nitric oxide, improving endothelial function and microcirculatory complications associated with diabetes.

Congestive Heart Failure

In a clinical study of 156 patients with congestive heart failure, 79 patients received 1.2-2 g berberine daily plus conventional medications, while 77 patients received placebo plus conventional medications, for eight weeks. Subjects in the berberine group had statistically significant improvements in cardiac function

(NYHA classification), six-minute walking test, left ventricular ejection fraction, dyspnea-fatigue indexes, resting blood pressure, and mortality (seven in the berberine group and 13 in the placebo group).

While we are not suggesting berberine to treat congestive heart failure, it is important to point out that berberine has shown to support a cardiovascular condition in which the thiazolidinediones have been implicated to cause.

Safety/Interactions

In a randomized, crossover study of healthy males, two weeks of berberine (300 mg three times daily) decreased the activity of the cytochrome p450 (CYP) enzymes CYP2D6, CYP2C9, and CYP3A4.42 Decreasing the activity of cytochrome p450 enzymes can slow the clearance of drugs metabolized by these enzymes, resulting in higher than expected blood levels. Berberine is contraindicated during pregnancy because it is thought to stimulate uterine contractions.

Conclusion

Berberine has been shown to offer benefits in the management of factors of metabolic syndrome in many ways. It can be used as a first line of nutritional therapy for clients who are border line, to those present with a number of different metabolic syndrome risk factors. Berberine also has been shown to be a suitable complimentary therapy to prescription medications where a practitioner is looking to enhance results while at the same time avoiding some side-effects which might result from medication therapy.

How to Recommend Berberine

In clinical studies it seems the threshold dosage for berberines' affects has been a minimum 1 gram daily. Where berberine has exhibited ability as a compliment to prescription medications, it is important to note that berberine does decrease activity of cytochrome p450, thus could possibly alter blood levels of influenced medications.

Below is a chart which highlight's both metabolic disorders/risk factors as well as common supplements used to support such conditions, either alone or as complimentary therapy. As you will see, Berberine plays a role in many different risk factors and conditions, and has been shown to be complimentary supportive in addition to medication and nutritional therapy.

Looking at the chart below, green represents primary nutrition supplement support which means that the supplement has shown sufficient results in regards to the condition or risk factor by itself. The purple color represents supplements of complementary support, ones which have not generally shown sufficient results as individual therapy.

Metabolic Disorder / Risk Factor Natural Supplement Chart

	Niacin	Berberine	Plant Sterols	Fish Oil	Chromium	Lipoic Acid	Co Q10	Carnitine
Raise HDL	✓			✓	✓			✓
Lower LDL	✓	✓	✓		✓			✓
Lower Total Cholesterol		✓	✓		✓			
Lower Triglycerides	✓	✓		✓	✓			✓
Lower Blood Press		✓		✓			✓	✓
Healthy Weight Mgmt		✓			✓	✓		✓
Blood Sugar/Insulin		✓		✓	✓	✓	✓	

Primary Support

Complimentary Support

TAKE CHARGE®

PROFESSIONAL OBESITY EDUCATION • HEALTHY LIFESTYLE STRATEGIES

WILL YOU ACCEPT THE TAKE CHARGE® CHALLENGE?

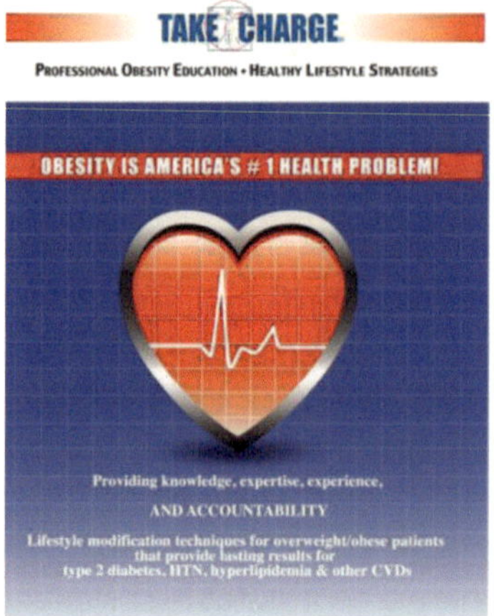

For a *minimum* of one year take the Money you are spending on Throw-Away-Advertising and invest it **in the Take Charge®** System. Let us show you how we can bring value to your specific situation.

ONLY $299.00 a month can add a service with a proven track record of improving ***both*** patient care and pharmacy profitability.

Now is the time to join us in implementing a system of treatment that can position you to ***both*** help your patients and revitalize your pharmacy practice by replacing lost reimbursement dollars.

Is your pharmacy prepared to work with ACO's?

ACCEPT THE CHALLENGE!

Call us at 800-782-3444 or email us at info@takechargerx.com for details and let Take Charge® do for you what it has done for hundreds of others!

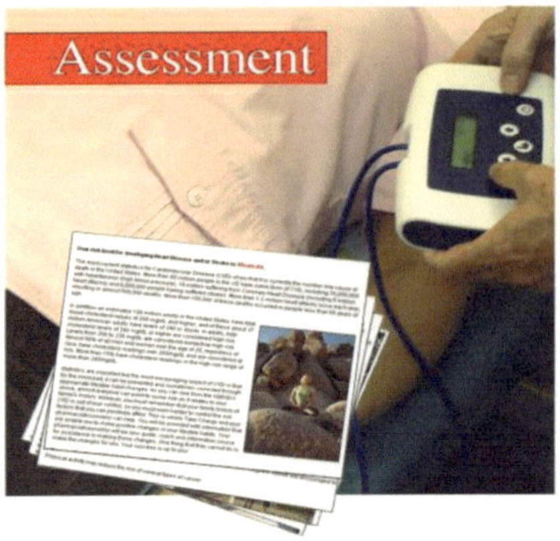

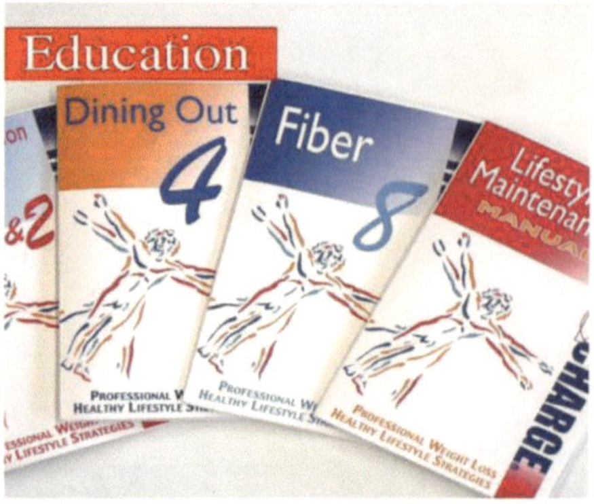

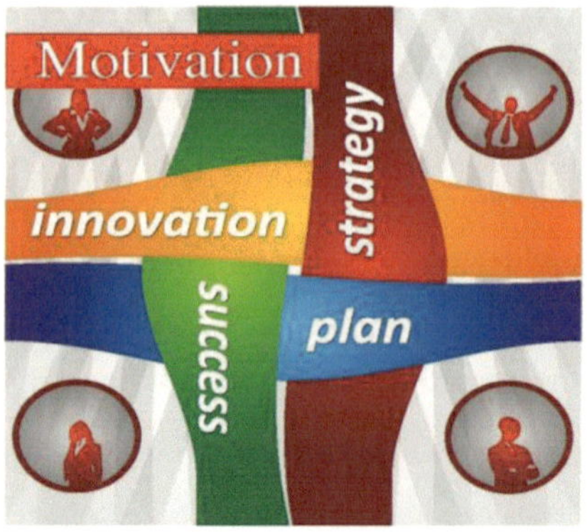

Homeopathy 101

How and why you should use homeopathy in your practice

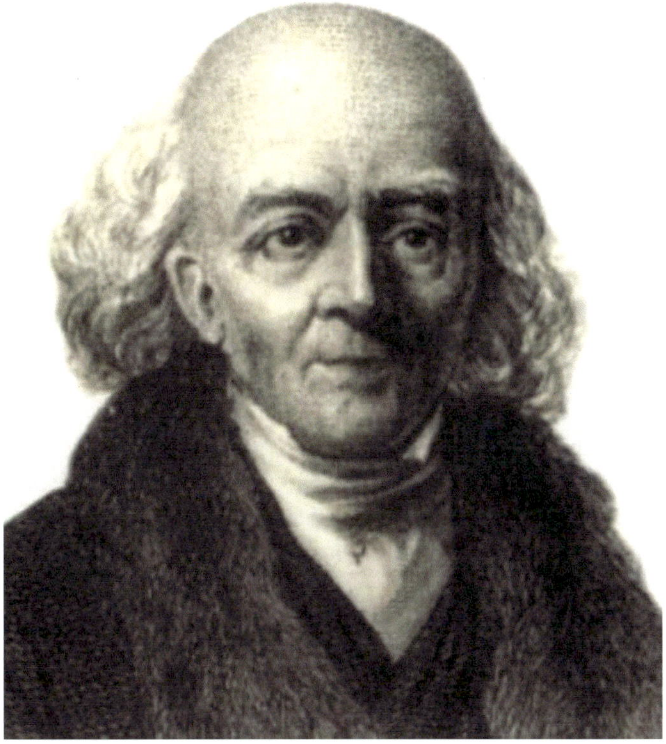

Samuel Hahnemann The Father of Homeopathy

When I was doing my clinical rounds for pharmacy at Hahnemann Hospital in Philadelphia, PA, curiously I never found much information on the teaching hospitals namesake...Samuel Hahnemann, the father of homeopathy. I understood that I was there for allopathic medicine, although even in 1994 I was searching for a more integrative approach and when I questioned my instructors if we would be learning anything in regards to homeopathy in the treatment of patient care, well, let's just say it fell on deaf ears.

> *"The highest ideal of therapy is to restore health rapidly, gently, permanently; to remove and destroy the whole disease in the shortest, surest, least harmful way, according to clearly comprehensible principles."*
>
> **Samuel Hahnemann**, Organon, 6'th ed.

The above statement by pharmacist and physician, Samuel Hahnemann, is the beauty of homeopathy. Homeopathy is an exceptionally safe and effective form of medicine that treats the whole individual, is applicable to all ages, and is tremendously underutilized in the United States.

Through his work Hahnemann created some core practices to homeopathy which are now regularly practiced in integrative medicine, such as recognizing that one's health is the result of numerous forces acting on the human body including; genetics, environment, hygiene, stress (mental, emotional, physical), diet, and exercise.

Samuel Hahnemann discovered homeopathy over 200 years ago with an experiment on himself. Though perfectly healthy at the time, he found that by giving himself repeated doses of cinchona bark (quinine), he brought on all the symptoms of a malaria attack -fever with heat and chills. Quinine was a treatment for malaria.

Hahnemann then experimented by diluting and then succussing a substance (shaking through striking the vial a number of times between numerical potencies). He realized that the potentised remedy was safer to use on the sick, and any unwanted side effects disappeared and the medicines were more effective.

Hahnemann tested 99 substances on himself and healthy volunteers known as Provers, keeping detailed accounts of his observations, thus leading him to be the first practitioner to implement complete case taking in his patient assessments. He then matched the tested substances to heal symptoms of his patients using the Law of Similars.

Law of Similars or "like cures like" states that all pharmacologically active substances create a characteristic set of symptoms when administered to healthy people. It then recognizes that all sick people display a set of symptoms that are characteristic of their disease. The conclusion is then made that the cure may be obtained by administering weak/infinitesimal doses of a substance whose experimental symptoms in healthy people are similar to symptoms displayed by the ill patient.

Due to the significance of dilution behind homeopathy, there is generally no fear of drug interactions, thus is safe to take in almost any situation, and often a suitable complement to prescription and nutrition therapy. Most homeopathic preparations are diluted down to the point where the active ingredients are no longer physically detectable.

The term homeopathy comes from two Greek words, *omia* (meaning "same"), and *pathos* (meaning "suffering"). What this means is that a homeopathic remedy is one that produces the same symptoms as those the sick person complains of, and in doing so sharply provokes the body into throwing them off.

Where the optimal choosing of a homeopathic medicine is based on a patient's mental, emotional and physical constitutional type as well as the totality of symptoms, let's take a look at some examples of homeopathic recommendations and ones symptoms based on the Law of Similars.

An individual who has been stung by a bee will experience pain and inflammation, and a stinging feeling. A remedy for this can be Apis mellifica, the honey bee.

Another example is for people who have trouble sleeping. The homeopathic of coffee, coffee cruda, can be a remedy of choice.

A common one used to help people alleviate hot flashes is lachesis mutas. Lachesis mutas is the homeopathic of the venom of a snake. What are the symptoms of a snake bite? Hot, burning, constricted feeling, just like a hot flash.

It is important to note that homeopathic preparations can be either over the counter or by prescription only.

Due to the fact that homeopathic remedies are closely controlled under the FDA, homeopathic preparations can actually make claims as to what they can treat, the opposite of nutritional supplements. For example if you were to pick up a tube of arnica you would see on the side that it says "Trauma, Bruises, and Muscle Soreness."

To hone in a step further, to make it easier to recommend homeopathic preparations, you can purchase what is known as a repertory. A repertory is an index of symptoms and systems of the body with remedies that affect the system listed under each heading.

For example, if I was to look up "Bronchitis" I would look for the exact symptoms the individual is experiencing. I dial into a symptom description that parallels that of the individuals such as "as symptoms get worse lying down or in stuffy rooms, cough is dry at night but loose in morning, lack of thirst." The remedy points to pulsatilla 6c.

Like nutrition, homeopathy is actually core to the practice of pharmacy. Most pharmacists in the 1800s and early 1900s were trained in compounding homeopathic/eclectic medicines.

Where homeopathy all but died out in the U.S. in the early 1900's it has been on a strong rebound in recent years. In the United States, of the people who try homeopathic agents, 84% say they would use them again.

In other countries through Europe homeopathy is the leading "alternative" treatment by physicians with growing numbers in the citizenry, and is even taught in medical schools. And despite homeopathy's impressive popularity in Europe, it is actually even more popular in India where over 100 million people depend solely on this form of medical care.

Homeopathy has a bright future in America, as it is the perfect complementary therapy to allopathic medicine and nutrition alike. Homeopathy has no known side-effects or interactions, can be used by any age group, even animals, and is very inexpensive, while paralleling the growing trend of individualized medicine.

Cosmeceutical Trends

The Intersection of Nutritional Supplements and Skin Care Cosmetics, From the Inside Out

By Amy G. Kress L.E.

Recently there has been increased attention paid to the physiological relationship between nutritional factors and the skin-ageing process. Corresponding to the trend, the healthy-ageing market has seen a robust growth in the so-called 'beauty from within' segment. This has been spurred by the demand of aging baby boomers and other health conscious individuals looking to do what it takes to remain or begin to look and feel young, healthy, and vital.

In the foreseeable future, more customers are expected to look for nutricosmetic foods and supplements that improve skin health. Companies are racing to develop healthy-ageing ingredients and products that can be either applied or consumed. A perfect example of this is food giant Coca Cola stepping into the functional beverage market partnering with pharmaceutical company Sanofi to launch a new line of beauty drinks known as Beautific Oenobiol.

As a pharmacist, you have the ability to meet your customers "where it hurts" and provide both functional and cosmetic solutions with the power of cosmeceuticals, while at the same time, supporting your bottom line.

In this issue I would like to highlight the benefits of collagen in cosmeceutical products, address how it helps from the beauty point of view, as well as share the other benefits collagen can provide, thus expanding your market.

Hormonal imbalance and hormonal exhaustion are epidemic in our society, and have far lasting effects on issues such as beauty, skin health, and overall wellbeing.

Think about all of the people who are walking around with subclinical or mismanaged hypothyroidism. These are the folks who might be ripe with low thyroid symptoms, but either due to improper assessment or inadequate testing, they fall through the cracks.

In the minds and words of your clients, what symptoms are they noticing with hypothyroidism? Hypothyroidism has many symptoms, and from a "how we are function-

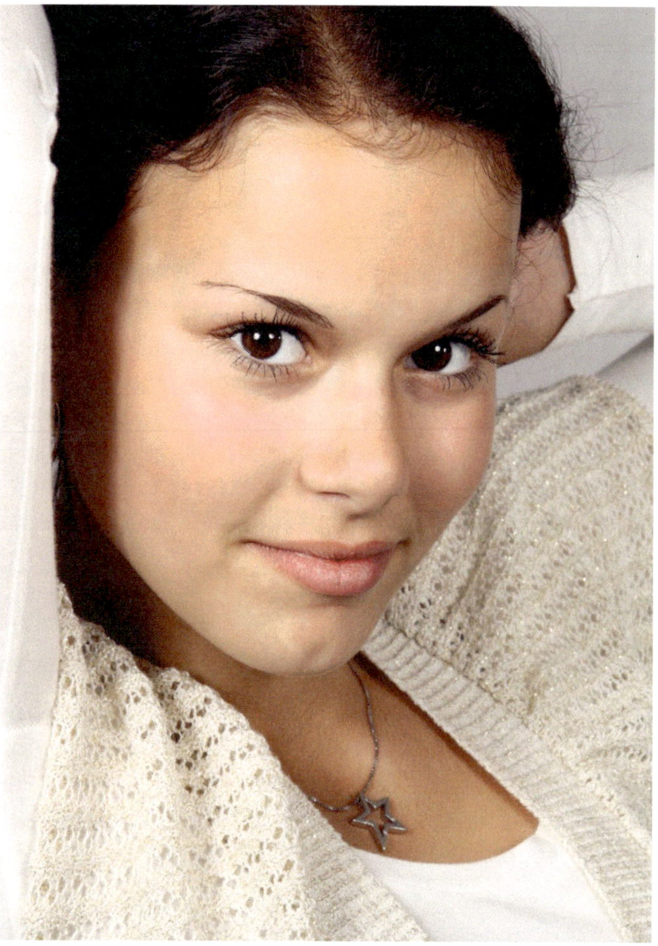

ing, feeling the pain and vanity" point of view, some of the most common complaints you will find in clients with hypothyroidism are dry skin, brittle hair and nails, fine lines and wrinkles, and joint pain and achiness.

How about people affected by mismanaged stress? Cortisol is a primary stress hormone and is considered "the enemy of collagen." When the two face off the result can be anything from joint pain to skin problems.

So...how can you help these folks with these painful, emotionally driven symptoms?

One of my favorite supplement ingredients is collagen; I find it answers many of the common problems clients complain of, many of them the middle aged female with improperly managed hypothyroidism and stress, that are tired and frustrated by their aches, pains, dry skin, fine lines and wrinkles.

While there are a number of different collagens on the market, I would like to share with you what the evidence and outcome base results are showing, and why this ingredient provides many applications in your practice.

Recently BioCell Technology announced publication of the first human skin study of BioCell Collagen® in the *Journal of Clinical Interventions in Aging*. This study enrolled 26 women between the ages of 35 to 59 which demonstrated the safety and significant efficacy of orally ingested BioCell Collagen in improving the visible signs of aging and dermal aging.

After 12 weeks, the subjects who were aged 35 to 59 years, showed a significant reduction of skin dryness/scaling (76 percent) and of fine lines and wrinkles (13.2 percent), as compared to baseline levels. The improved appearance was explained by internal metabolic shift in the dermis, leading to an increase in collagen content (3.5 percent) and in blood microcirculation (15 percent). As a result, a majority of the study participants experienced a remarkable improvement in skin texture, together with hydration, reduced scaling and improved blood microcirculation.

Beyond Beauty

Let's face it; many other challenges come with aging in addition to fine lines and wrinkles. Joint achiness is often an issue, whether it is a side-effect of hormonal imbalance or exhaustion, or the bone structure feeling its years. Collagen preparations such as BioCell Collagen have shown to offer additional joint motility and comfort in addition to the benefits of health skin.

Osteoporosis is another area where collagen supplementation could provide a benefit. Collagen is a strong, flexible and fibrous protein that gives bones a framework for strength and flexibility. As bones loose this framework, they have the potential to lose flexibility increasing potential to crack, shatter and break. This has led to research in the area of collagen for bone support, and the development of a calcium and collagen complex known as KoACT.

KoACT is a calcium collagen chelate designed to improve bone strength. KoACT delivers both calcium and bone collagen at the same time and was shown to increase femur bone strength 9.9% more than calcium alone in a university study. This is important to note, knowing the risk factors spontaneous fracture caused by long term use of bisphosphonate medications.

How can you see collagen fitting into your nutritional arsenal? Above we have outlined a few, very common disease states and symptoms this nutritional powerhouse can help to support.

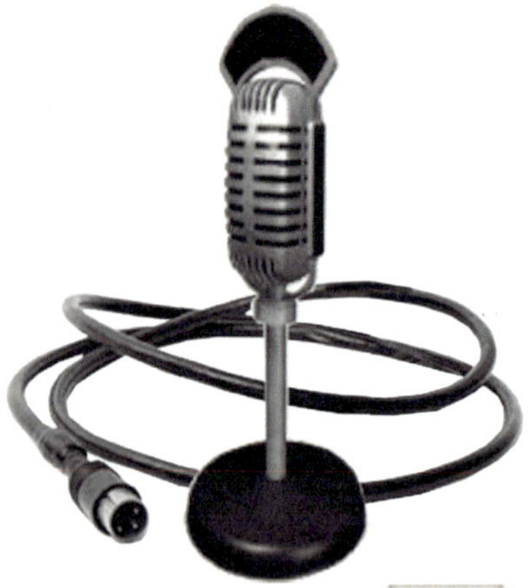

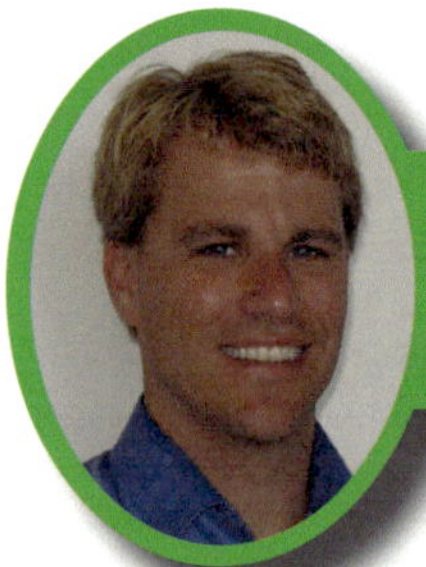

Ask The Marketing Pharmacist:

"I am opening a new pharmacy; we will be compounding, selling regular prescriptions, and pharmaceutical grade nutrition.

How do I set myself apart from the competition?"

By Robert B Kress RPh

I love this question, because not only does it apply to someone just opening a new pharmacy or any business for that matter- this applies to everyone, regardless of how long you have been in business or even how successful you are.

Let's face it, we are not taught this stuff in pharmacy school, so I want to share with you **the 5 part backbone** to ANY marketing plan, these are the foundational elements; Category, Position, USP, Elevator Speech, Brand Personality.

First, let's talk about positioning. One of the greatest books I have read in marketing is Positioning, by Reiss and Trout. I suggest everyone to read this book; it is an invaluable resource and explains perfectly how to be the #1 in your category.

Category and Position

Your customers think in ways of categories, and so should you about your business. Your goal is to be number 1 in your category, and if you cannot, then it's up to you to create a new category and own it. Categories are like place holders, quick to go to answers in our instant gratification society- and this realization keeps getting more and more important as people are continually bombarded with more and more information on a daily basis.

So, when someone says- "how do I stop these hot flashes" whether they are saying this to themselves or asking a friend- you want the automatic answer to be YOU. You are the category they immediately think of and go to so they can begin to solve their problem.

Picture an icon on your desk top that you click on to get on the internet, categories are short-cuts to make people's lives easier.

What category are you in? And do you own it? Here are some examples of categories in pharmacy, and the difference with each one is the offerings, and remember, everything you offer, communicate it as a benefit- that's what people are looking for. And even if you are new to something which you offer- make it your goal to become the obvious expert in your market.

Pharmacy category examples: Compounding only, Compounding only and nutrition, Traditional, compounding and nutrition, Traditional only, Nutritional Pharmacy, etc.

Say for instance that you are a complete traditional, compounding and nutritional pharmacy, and there is major competition in your area. Right now you are not #1 and becoming #1 in this area seems like a long haul. Then, create your own category in your market.

Maybe you can Zen things up, add a tea room, bring in an integrative practitioner, massage therapist, - closer to a health center. Or you can focus on one area big time, maybe nutrition, and where you offer everything that the competition does, you do this one thing better than anyone.

In either case, claim this unmarked category and own it.

So, how do you let people know this is your category and you are the only choice?

USP (Unique Selling Proposition)

I came across this need in my own pharmacy. We had a sign that said, Nutritional Pharmacy...people came in asking "what is it exactly that you do?", and it took me a little bit to dial in my response... which can save you a ton of time, aggravation, and prevent customers from never knowing ALL that you offer.

USP stands for Unique Selling Proposition. Your USP describes why someone would want to shop with you above and beyond the competition. Remember, speak benefits.

Ex- *"We get you feeling great again through customized health solutions to fit your unique needs."*

Let's take this out of the pharmacy realm and give you an example which literally was the catapult to put Domino's Pizza on the map, ***"fresh, hot pizza to your door in 30 minutes or less or its free."*** They have since changed it due to a series of lawsuits related to traffic accidents of drivers rushing to make the delivery.

Let's deconstruct this USP:

- **Fresh** - customer benefit – who wants old and stale?
- **Hot** - customer benefit – hot is how most pizza eat pizza, no need to re-heat and wait, begin enjoying immediately.
- **Pizza** – the targeted result, what you are getting - it's not a vague "meal" or "hunger satisfied"
- **Delivered to your door** - customer benefit- I don't have to travel to get it, or make it, I can do other stuff while waiting for it, they do all the work.
- **In 30 minutes or less** - a specific promise. You can be rest assured that in a specified amount of time your desire will be satisfied.
- **Or it's free** - the guarantee- We are so confident that your desire will be satisfied how and when we say it will, and if not, it's yours free.

Elevator Speech

Basically, if you had just 2 minutes to convince someone to shop at your store while riding in an elevator, what would you say?

Ex- *"Not everyone is the same and we believe that health care should not be a one size fits all approach. We integrate the best of age old traditions and modern day discoveries to reduce side-effects, dependence on prescription drugs, while helping our customers sleep better, have more energy, reduce hot flashes, lose weight and more. Since the nutrition and cosmetic industries have few regulation's we only carry high quality products which are free of the toxic tagalongs found in many supplements and skin care products- all at great value."*

Brand Personality

Brand personality is how you are perceived and is the culmination of your beliefs, values, and your back story.

What do you stand for? What drives you? Why is it you do what you do? As a pharmacist, is it to help your customers in all matters of health? Is it to show your clients on how to be an advocate for their own health? Is it to provide people with information and products which are seldom offered to them? Maybe it's to provide the highest quality of products and service, second to none?

What you stand for can also be described as your values. Values are- well, what you find value in. Basically what makes you feel great and what makes you feel bad.

For example, it makes me feel really bad when I see animals being abused or without a home, or a handicap child- I find it unjust, thus justice is a core value of mine. Another would be the overly biased chemical and surgery based medical system, where many people are told just to accept their state of health. This is where I really value vitality, because I know we can attain it, and it energizes me to help people find it.

This leads to an example of a core value which makes you feel good. I love helping people feel better, solving problems, finding self-empowerment in their health. This makes me feel fulfilled, yet other strong values.

Do you think a customer or client would like to have someone in their corner who will do all they can to fight for them, drive them towards vitality, not hindered or held down by illness, while guiding them to feeling self-empowered about being healthy? Especially in the face of injustice or dealing with a medical system providing few answers, I think here you have a customer for life.

So now that we know what we stand for, you need a back story to support it, one that is congruent with what you stand for. The backstory is what you share with people when you introduce you and your practice; it's the reason why a local paper or media outlet would want to do a story about you. One important thing...you want to add in a hook. A hook is what makes the backstory interesting, it's what makes people want to learn more.

My personal back story and what I stood for was (is),

> *"I was fed up with seeing the merry-go-round of prescriptions, and medications being used to treat side-effects of other medications so I decided I had to make a change. My wife and I wanted to provide a place for people to go where they could talk with a health care professional who knows the risks, benefits and limitations of both prescription drugs and natural medicines. This is why I have created my own pharmacy to provide a balance, and inform people on what they need to know in seeking the best for their health and to really help people feel better, often after years of forgetting what it feels like to feel great"*

Now, one can certainly add a more impactful hook to this story. For instance, I have known many integrative practitioners who have a 'reason why' they went this direction in medicine. Where mine was 'being fed up with the model I was practicing under', there are folks who have had life altering experiences, leading them in this direction.

There you have it, now time to put together your **5 part backbone** to your marketing.

Action Plan Steps- Answer these questions:

1. What is your category?
2. What position do you hold?
3. Are you #1? If not, can you create a new category and what would it be?
4. What is your USP?
    a. What is Your Elevator Speech?
    b. What is Your Brand Personality? (Beliefs, Values, Back Story)

Looking for someone who has your back, a soundboard to bounce your marketing ideas off of, a resource for marketing content, nutritional and creative marketing coaching and to ask questions, go to www.functionalpharmacy.com

Made in the USA
Monee, IL
05 November 2026

67953742R00031